THE

FBI

FIT BODY INITIATIVE

To David & Brenda

All the best for your

"New" fit future

Steve

APR 2009

90 DAYS TO A FITTER, HEALTHIER, YOU

THE FBI

FIT BODY INITIATIVE

STEVE HALLS

LEANMARKETING™
★PRESS★

First Published In Great Britain 2006
by Lean Marketing Press
www.BookShaker.com

Typeset in Trebuchet

WARNING

This book is not intended to be an alternative to personal, professional medical advice. If you have any concerns about your current level of health you should consult your doctor before partaking in any new or vigorous training or making big diet changes. While the information in this book is believed to be accurate at the time of going to press neither the author nor the publisher can accept any legal responsibility for errors or omissions which may be made.

Dedicated to...

My darling wife Marie who has given her unconditional love and support throughout. I love you.

My clients, past and present. Your efforts and achievements are where I gather my enthusiasm and enjoyment, Thanks for that.

CONTENTS

ACKNOWLEDGEMENTS

Tony Burgess and Julie French - Directors of the Academy of High Achievers (Aha!) - for their constant inspiration and for giving me the opportunity to work with so many amazing people.

Debbie Jenkins and Joe Gregory - publishers at www.bookshaker.com - without whose help this project would have not got off the ground.

Stew Evans - for asking me to do a quick 90 one liner tips that sort of manifested into the book it is today.

FOREWORD

Why do today what you can put off doing until tomorrow?

If you're exhausted by the thought of having to walk to the TV to change channels because you can't find the remote control.

If your friends somehow always manage to look fitter, healthier and slimmer than you, and you think "ah well... I'll just have to learn to live with it".

If you've ever had someone tell you (in an overly-enthusiastic way) that "you can become addicted to exercise and you'll learn to love it", but you felt like ramming their dumb bells where the sun don't shine because a) you simply didn't believe that what they were saying was possible and b) you didn't need a smarmy athlete in your face, pointing out your fitness failures!!

... Then you're in the shoes which I've now, thankfully, vacated! The man to thank is Steve Halls.

I'd spent at least five years B.S. in this state of mind: five years B.S. being five years Before Steve. Having trained as a dancer for about twelve years, it was a shock to find myself in a situation where I had no interest in exercise at all. I would happily have dropped a hammer onto my own toe to avoid being dragged to the gym; and who needs Lycra, sweat and breathlessness anyway? Euchh! Times change, don't they? A job, more responsibilities, not enough hours in the day, so exercise is thrown out of the window. It takes effort, it's expensive to join a gym, and it's selfish because it's something which only benefits you, rather than everyone else around you. From page one of this book, you'll find out just how misguided those feelings are.

As an Army veteran, he'll hate me for saying this, but Steve is my Fairy Godmother: only magic could have made me realise that spending a little time each week, pushing myself to feel pain in muscles I didn't even know I had, could make me feel so good! Steve is firm but fair and always manages to find something more in you, when you feel there's nothing more you can give: he's the only person I know who has the humour to make me laugh whilst doing press ups and has taught me that looking after myself needn't be hell.

Before you think of me as the "smarmy athlete" trying to tell you how great exercise is, let me say that I'm no athlete. It is an effort, it is hard work, but I would never look back because the positives far outweigh the negatives. Since Steve took me under his wing, I'm fitter, healthier, slimmer, and above all, happier. Finding a small amount of time for exercise has given me more energy, and more importantly, given me my confidence back.

You have to want to do the training, because it's not easy, and anyone can find an excuse to bail out. The fact that you're reading this book is proof enough that you're thinking about your health, and believe me, if Steve can help me, he can help you too. No gyms, no Lycra, no looking back. Squats, Sit Ups and Steve Halls... it's the perfect combination, so what are you waiting for? COME ON!

Janine Machin
BBC Radio Stoke

INTRODUCTION

This is a 90 day fitness program with a difference. With nutritional, lifestyle and exercise information, tips and a call to action, it is a comprehensive life-changing tool.

It is suitable for all people regardless of age or ability. It has been designed to build up gradually in order to slowly introduce exercise into your daily life. As the course is progressive it is therefore important that all the days are done in order. Like any course, you only get out what you put in. If just by buying this book you are inspired to take action, then imagine how great it's going to feel when you've completed it fully.

I can promise that if you give 100% you will see and feel a difference. A training partner or "buddy" can also help to keep you on track, so if you would like to get in touch with someone to hold you accountable in return for your support to them, contact me via my website www.stevehalls.co.uk

I look forward to working with you for the next 3 months!

#1. KNOW WHERE YOU ARE NOW

To reach a particular destination in life we might use a plan or a map to help us to get there. To use a map you need to know not only your required destination but also your starting point. This applies too in your health and fitness plan. The first day is all about finding out where you are now. It is important to know exactly where you are now in respect to health and fitness.

To achieve this you need to take certain measurements. Some of them require specialist equipment found in a Gym, The Doctors or from a Personal Trainer, whereas some tests can be obtained very easily in the comfort of your own home.

Measurements to take are Blood Pressure, Height, Weight, Body Fat % and Resting Heart Rate. Using a tape measure get the circumferential measurements from your hips and waist. These serve as a benchmark and are to be repeated at 6 weekly intervals to monitor your progress. You must take all readings accurately so you can replicate the tests.

You might also want to have a photo of you taken to create your own "Before and After" picture to show others the great success that you will have achieved having completed and applied the course. This may feel awkward at first but just imagine the impact it will have on you as you start to make those desired changes.

My Vital Statistics	
Blood Pressure	...
Height	...
Weight	...
Body Fat %	...
Resting Heart Rate	...
Hip Measurement	...
Waist Measurement	...

COME ON!

- Arrange to have all the measurements taken.
- If you cannot do them all today, do as many as you can so you have at least started.
- Use the template provided or make up your own accordingly.
- Do that photo shoot, you'll be so glad that you did.
- Suggested kit for training is a good pair of running/cross trainers, Skipping Rope, set of dumbbells, a cushioned mat and for the ladies a good supportive (sports) bra. These are not essential as an alternative could be used.

#2. KNOW WHERE YOU'RE GOING

Achievable and realistic goals in the fitness world act as a motivating factor and a positive direction for your training. They should also stretch you. An easy goal is pointless.

By all means let your mind think big but a goal that is clearly out of your physical range will only act as a de-motivating tool. For example, if you're a non runner today, setting a goal of running (without stopping) a double marathon next week would not be the best idea that you would have had. Break that major goal into smaller goals so you have an easier target to aim at. Build in a purposeful training regime with a realistic time frame and you stand an excellent chance of succeeding.

We will be building a general training regime day by day, but for specialist stuff you may need to get in touch with me outside of this course.

COME ON!

- Write down your ultimate health and fitness goal or goals.
- Break them down into smaller chunks so that you have targets in front of you that are easier to attain, this will help to keep you motivated.
- Put your goals somewhere that you will see them daily. Look at them, believe them and do something every day to move you closer to them.

In the next section we will look at a simple warm up routine to mobilise all the joints in the body ready for exercise.

#3. MOBILISE ALL THE JOINTS

Warming up is an essential part of the workout. This raises the heart rate and gets the blood pumping faster into the muscles that are being asked to work. It also prevents injury. Because of the complex nature of the warm up we will split the process in two.

Today we will learn a general mobility routine to loosen off all the joints from top to bottom. All the joints in the body stiffen up through age and over night to a lesser degree. Each person will experience a different degree of discomfort first thing in the morning. Mobilising the joints can alleviate this stiffness. Movement of your joints will stimulate your natural lubrication (synovial fluid) within them.

This mobility routine can be carried out either standing or sitting with a few slight differences depending on your particular health issues.

THE ROUTINE: (Repeat all these actions at least 8 times before moving on to the next warm-up exercise)

- Swivel your head from side to side as if you were indicating a big "no".
- Move your head up and down (not too far up) as if indicating a big "yes".
- Tilt your head to the side by trying to put your ear on your shoulder then repeat on the other side.
- Shrug your shoulders (remember your early days when you were naughty, who broke the window? A shrug of the shoulders was a natural reaction) then push them as far down as you can.
- Bring your shoulders forward then push them to the rear.
- Roll your shoulders forward, making the circles as big as possible. Then roll them backwards.
- Bend down to each side in turn reaching down the side of your legs with your hands. Reach a little further with each bend. If you're sat down reach down the sides of the chair towards the floor.

- Put your arms in front of your body and twist your torso from side to side. Start off gradually and then reach round as far as you can go each time you twist.
- Lift your lower arms to your shoulders bending them at the elbows.
- Clasp your hands together and rotate the wrists in both directions.
- Swivel the hips in a circular motion. First one way and then the other. Keep your head and shoulders still during the movement. *
- Tilt the pelvis to the front and then the rear. As you thrust out to the front be careful whom you make eye contact with. It could shape your future life forever. *
- Bend the knees forward and back if you are standing. Slowly does it, ensuring that your knees do not travel further forward than your toes. Place your hands on your knees as you do this. If you're sat down, lift one leg at a time until the leg is straight out in front of you. Bend it back down, change legs and repeat.
- Make small circles with the knees still keeping hold of the knees. Repeat the movement in the opposite direction. *
- Rotate the ankle joint in both directions one foot at a time. If standing place a foot behind you and rotate the foot pivoting on your toes. If sat down, lift your leg in front of you.

*Means, that if you are sat down you will not be able to carry out this particular mobility exercise.

This routine should only last for about 5 minutes at the most.

COME ON!

- Practise the mobility routine.
- Use music if you want. It usually helps people to get in an exercise mood. I find that Bryan Adams' "Summer of 69" the ideal song to do the routine to.
- Get into a habit of doing this small routine every day to get the body moving.

#4. WATER WORKS

Water is the king of all drinks. It is pure and nutritionally sound, essential for vitality and the one small thing that can radically change your life.

As a general guideline, most adults should be drinking at least 2 litres of water per day. This is a minimum requirement for everyday intake. If you exercise a lot or sweat profusely, then you'll need to increase this amount. If you do not drink this amount now, then you will probably find difficulty in swallowing that much in a day. Have a strategy. Put small bottles around the house, in the car etc so when you see them you take a drink from them. Drink before you're thirsty.

Our body is made up of 70% water, and the water we drink is required to replace cells that die off through natural wastage. Without the water, we cannot replace the cells that we lose.

If you're thirsty you're already partially dehydrated which causes a lack of performance. Stave off the ageing process and start drinking that water now.

COME ON!

- Keep a track of how much water you drink in a day.
- Pour out 2 litres (roughly 4 pints) and make sure that by the end of the day you are close if not over your recommended allowance.
- Gradual improvement is of course accepted, as sometimes it is not that easy to consume this much at first.

Get that wet stuff down your neck; you will really notice the difference!

#5. WARMING UP THE MUSCLES

After mobilising all the joints, it is imperative to warm up the muscles before you do any strenuous exercise. The harder the workout, the harder the intensity of the warm-up you should be doing.

Why do we warm up?

By raising the body temperature gradually, warm-up activities provide various physiological benefits. These are:

- Raises your core body temperature, which causes vasodilatation (widening of the blood vessels). This increases the blood supply and provides more oxygen to your tissues and working muscles.
- Your muscles and other connective tissues contract, relax and stretch more readily when they are warm.
- Metabolic activity in your muscle tissue is stimulated.
- The viscosity within your muscles is reduced, which allows smoother and more efficient contractions with less resistance.
- Your muscles are able to exert greater power under sub-maximal loads.
- Your nervous impulses travel more rapidly. This applies to motor and sensory nervous pathways, improving general proprioceptive activity (the information supplied by receptors in the body that tells the brain the state of the body at any given time).
- The response of your heart to more strenuous exercise is improved significantly.
- Mental preparation is an important factor in the warm-up or rehearsal effect.

Start with the general mobility exercise to loosen off all the joints from head to toe as normal.

Now you want to carry out some cardio-vascular exercise at a slower than normal pace gradually increasing the intensity. Types of cardio you could do are jogging, skipping, rowing, cycling, step machine etc.

If you're going to do a resistance (weights etc) session, your first set should be carried out using light weights.

COME ON!

- Here's your chance to put the mobility routine together with your warm-up.
- Put your favourite upbeat music on if appropriate and get stuck in.
- Mobility should take about 5 minutes and warm-up about 10 minutes.

Come on then, let's raise that pulse and get out of breath!

#6. COOL-DOWN

Just as you gradually increase the amount of work prior to strenuous exercise (your warm-up), so it makes sense to gradually decrease the amount of work following a "training session". This tapering off is called "cooling down" or "warming down".

Following intense activity, your blood has been diverted to your working muscles and there is a tendency for your blood to "pool" in the extremities, especially in your legs. Light rhythmical activity involving the muscle groups used in the exercise session should be used in this cool-down period, which often consists of the same exercises used for the warm-up. This will aid venous return (the blood returning) to the heart and help prevent pooling and consequent dizziness and nausea. These low intensity exercises not only disperse the lactic acid present but also prevent further build up of lactic acid.

Stretching activities during the warm-down would also seem to prevent muscle soreness following exercise. We will be looking at general stretching techniques throughout the book as the muscles are worked. Gradually bringing the body back to normal also helps psychological wind-down and promotes mental relaxation at the end of the exercise session, allowing time to consider the feeling of satisfaction and benefit that the exercise has given you.

COME ON!

- Practice firstly your warm-up routine including your mobility.
- Then perform your "Cool-Down" by gradually decreasing the intensity of the exercise.
- Carry out some light stretches of the muscles that you've just used.

Wallow in your great feeling

#7. EAT A BALANCED DIET

A balanced diet consists of roughly 20% Protein, 60% Carbohydrate and 20% Fat. It also ensures the correct Minerals and Vitamins are present.

This is a general requirement for most people, which may need tweaking if you're training for something sports specific. It is important to know why you must eat a balanced diet as this helps you to appreciate the value of the foods that we eat.

Protein has two major functions in the body; Structural and Functional. The structural side will build all that we see from muscles to bones etc. Whereas the functional side will be responsible for things like hormones, immune system and digestive enzymes; things that we don't see.

Carbohydrate is the body's preferred source of fuel. Without sufficient fuel you will feel lethargic and may experience a lack of concentration.

Fat protects the organs of the body. It also coats the nerves in a myelin sheath. It is also a reserve source of fuel for the body to utilise.

We will cover these in more detail later on in the book.

Below is an example of the breakdown of food that I would normally have for my breakfast. The figures are obtained from the packaging of the products. 1 gram of protein = 4 calories, 1 gram of carbohydrate = 4 calories and 1 gram of fat = 9 calories.

Item	Quantity	Protein	Carbs	Fat	Calories
Oats	75g	8.8g	51.0g	5.4g	288
Milk	100g	3.2g	4.8g	3.9	66
Toast x 2	100g	18.3	82.8	4.9g	428
Butter	10g	0.04g	0g	8.0g	72
Banana	100g	1.2g	23.2g	0.3g	95
TOTAL	-	31.54g	161.8g	22.5g	949

As you can see, my breakfast is a balanced blend of foods coming from all three sources. If you think that it's a lot of calories, my daily intake is over 4500.

COME ON!

- Look in your cupboards, fridge, freezer etc. and see what type of foodstuffs that you have.
- Identify, using the label whether the food is rich in protein, carbohydrate or fat.
- Plan to balance your cupboards with the 20-60-20 formula over your next few shopping trips.

#8. KEEP A FOOD DIARY

Keep a record of your intake. Everything that passes your lips should be recorded, as it will have calorific content. This enables you to make changes in your diet if they are required. You can't change something that you don't know about because you might change the wrong thing and make it worse.

Use the template provided on the next page or make your own and get used to weighing your food as you prepare it. This might sound a chore at first, but it does get easier the more you get used to it. For example, we normally pour out the same amount of cereal in our bowl everyday without weighing it. We also generally pour on the same amount of milk. Therefore by measuring it once and sticking to the portions we will know how much we are consuming.

It is better to eat first and analyse after rather than tallying up as you go through the day. This prevents you getting to the stage where you are in a pickle over what to have in your evening meal that is a certain calorific value.

Eat, Enjoy, Reflect, Analyse and then make the necessary changes if any are required.

COME ON!

- Make copies of the food diary template on the next page and start your diary from tomorrow.
- Be strict at first and you will soon get a good idea of what you're putting into your body on a daily basis.

We will look at what you're entitled to eat tomorrow.

FOOD DIARY TEMPLATE

Item	Quantity	Protein	Carbs	Fat	Calories

#9. KNOW WHAT YOU'RE ENTITLED TO

We've already mentioned about what is a simple balanced diet is, so using the percentages 20% Protein, 60% Carbohydrate and 20% fat we will work out what the body requires daily by grams.

- Take your weight in kg
- Multiply that by the number by grams of protein you require. This number ranges from 1 gram which is a sedentary person through 1.5 grams, which would be 3 hard sessions a week to 2.5 grams which is the maximum used by a serious power lifter.
- As the body needs the same amount of fat the numbers are the same.
- Carbohydrate required is 3 times that of protein therefore multiply the figure for protein by 3.

Here's an example: A typical man weighing 65kg with a sedentary lifestyle will require 65 grams (65 x 1) of protein, 65 grams (65 x 1) of fat and 195 (65 x 1 x 3) grams of carbs a day. A man weighing the same but who works out 3 times a week would require 97.5 grams (65 x 1.5) of protein, 97.5 grams (65 x 1.5) of fat and 292.5 grams (65 x 1.5 x 3) of carbs a day.

You now have the daily allowance for your fuel in grams. This can be turned into calories if desired by multiplying protein and carbohydrate by 4 and fat by 9.

COME ON!

- Using the method shown in the example, work out your own daily fuel allowance.
- Start to use correct portion sizes to match your requirements.

#10. YOUR FIRST CARDIO VASCULAR SESSION

Cardio Vascular training improves the functioning of your heart and lungs or the engine room of your body. It also improves the way that your oxygenated blood from the engine room gets round the body to the various muscles. Your Heart is a muscle and can be developed like all other muscles by pushing it out of its "comfort zone", which we talk about in depth on another day.

If you get out of breath, you are pushing yourself, which is a good indication that you are doing good work. Start off your Cardio-vascular training by walking, jogging or running. This will depend on where you are at with your fitness at this moment in time. The principle is the same throughout though. A simple program could consist of a 30-minute run/walk. Warm up the muscles gradually then do a timed effort. Turn round and come back again. Record the distance (use a landmark etc) and try to beat this the next time you go.

I prefer to run a straight course rather than a circuit. Purely a personal choice based on if you run out to a point in your best time, no matter how you feel, you have to get back to the start. Therefore there is no short cut or easy way out. Encouraging you to do a bit more work than you probably wanted to. This takes you out of your comfort zone.

After working the leg muscles, it is important to "stretch off" to avoid muscle soreness. Stretch off the leg muscles as shown in the photos...

FBI Quadriceps Stretch

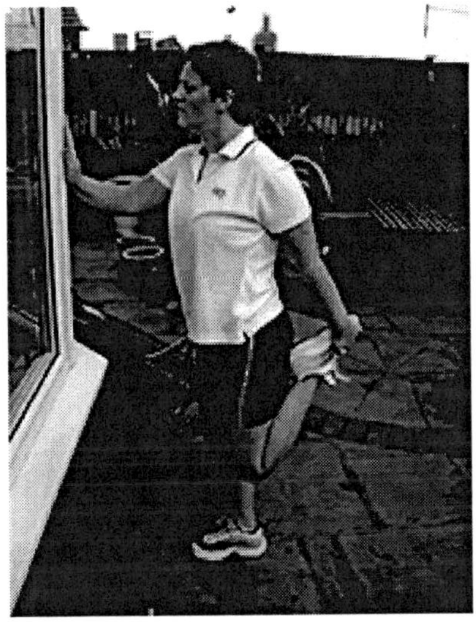

Bring your heel to your bum, keeping your knees together.

FBI Hamstrings Stretch

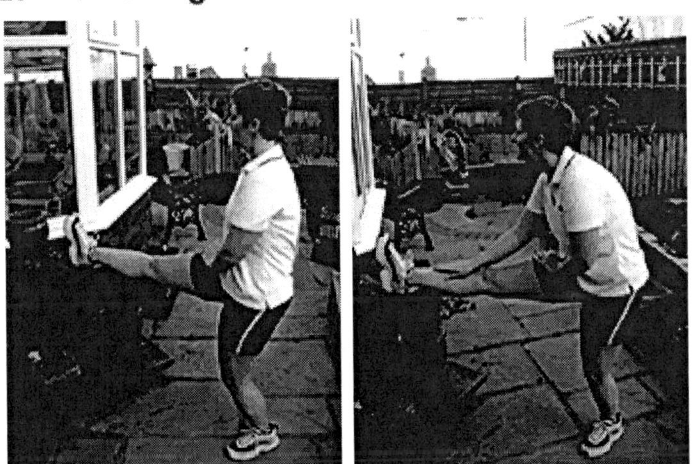

Place your outstretched leg on a bench. Lean forward from the waist until you feel a stretch on the back of the leg.

FBI Calf Stretch

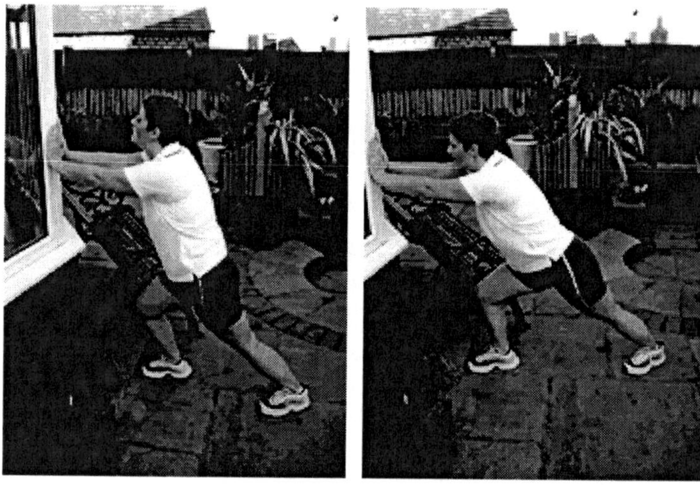

Put one leg behind the other and lean forwards using a support if necessary. Put your rear heel to the floor and feel the stretch in your rear calf.

COME ON!

- Find a safe route where you can walk, jog or run. A treadmill in the gym is acceptable but nothing beats the great outdoors.
- Do your mobility routine and warm up the muscles by steady walking for 5 minutes.
- Then walk/jog/run with a purpose (get a sweat on) for 10 minutes and remember how far you get.
- Turn round and come back again.
- Cool down and stretch off the muscles in your legs for 5 minutes.
- Record the distance.

#11. INCREASE YOUR LEAN MUSCLE

Lean muscle is the calorie burner within the body. The more lean muscle, the more calories you will burn on a daily basis even when you are at rest.

To increase lean muscle tissue, start to work the muscles in such a way that you are working them outside their comfort zone. This makes the body adapt and therefore change.

Start off by performing Squats. This is a great calorie burner as it is a large muscle group that you are working. In fact it is the largest muscle group in the body and will therefore burn you the most calories when worked. It can easily be done in the comfort of your own home without the prying eyes of strangers if you are the shy type. To carry out this exercise use a chair or bench behind you. Go to sit down on the bench making sure that your knees don't go forward of your toes. As your bum touches the bench, stand back up again.

FBI **Squats**

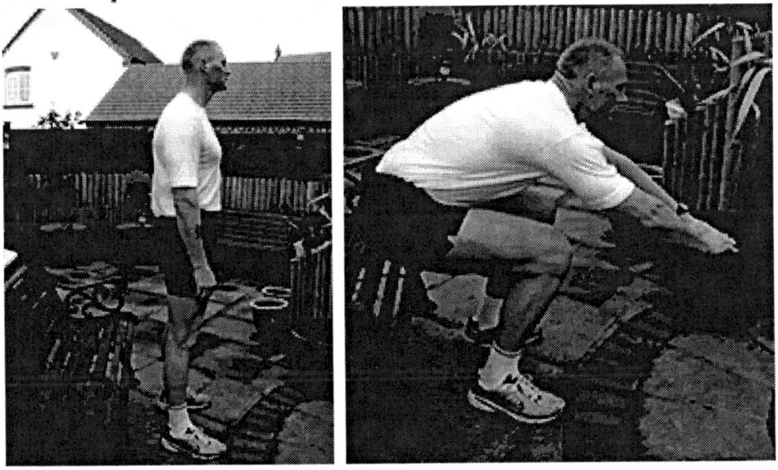

How easy is that? It is probably the most effective single exercise in this whole course and on top of that it is truly functional, as we sit down and stand up many times naturally every day.

COME ON!

- Start off by doing 10 repetitions of this exercise.
- Then it's time to make a commitment.
- Do 10 every time you go to sit down at home.

This habit alone will make a difference, I promise!

#12. ILLEGAL DRUGS AND POTIONS

It is always inappropriate for you to use illegal drugs to get the body shape you require.

Everything is possible with a good diet and the correct training regime so there is never an excuse for cheating. Pills and potions that promise the world do not work. The body thrives on "Good Fuel, Good Exercise and Good Company". So give the body what it needs and be prepared to give yourself time to achieve the changes. Some people expect changes to occur overnight but in health and fitness, progress occurs gradually.

It is hard to believe that some people find it so important to try and get quick results that they jeopardise their life for it. Drug abuse whether in sport or "recreational" is seriously damaging to the health of both your mind and body.

COME ON!

- Time for your second cardio session.
- Go for another walk/jog /run and record your progress.
- Let's get past your previous distance in the timed section.

Remember: Keep it clean - Keep it lean!

#13. ALWAYS TRAIN BIG MUSCLE GROUPS BEFORE SMALL ISOLATED MUSCLES

When carrying out resistance training (weights) always tire out the big muscle groups first before you train the smaller isolated muscles. This can prevent injuries occurring in the smaller muscles.

Examples of this are Lat Pulldown before Bicep Curls and Press-ups before Tricep Press.

We'll look at all these exercises in future lessons.

Today's exercise is the Press-up.

Your current strength level will determine the kind of press-up you will start off doing.

FBI Box Press-up

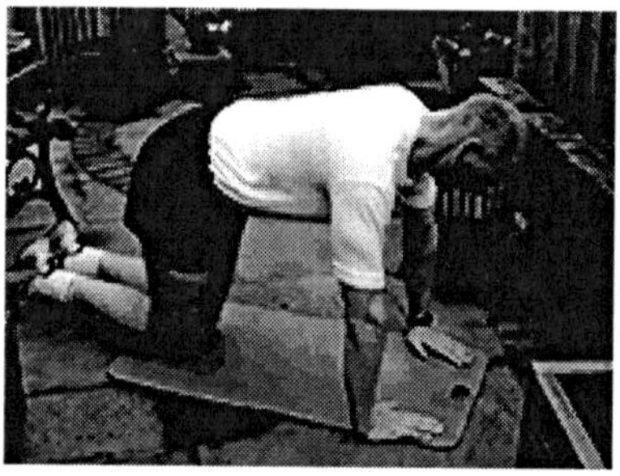

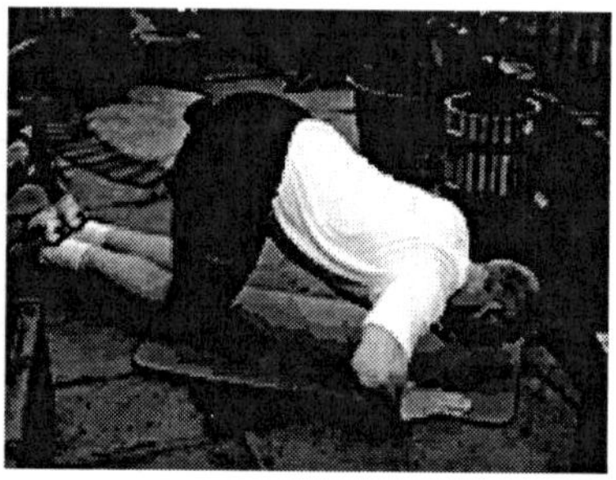

The easiest is the Box Press-up:

1. Adopt a position on all fours with your hands slightly more than shoulder width apart.
2. Lower the chest down to the floor and return again to the start.
3. Always breathe out when you do the work part of the exercise. In this case it is when you push back up to the starting position.

FBI 3/4 Press-up

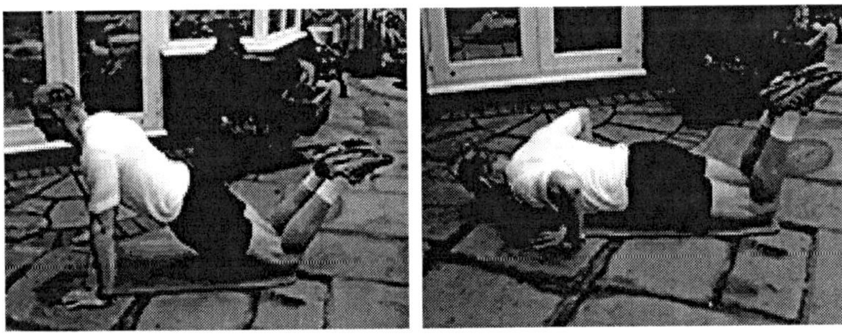

If you're **feeling stronger:**

1. Start off lying on your front, with your legs bent at the knees.
2. With your hands below your shoulders push up and pivot on the fleshy part of your knees.
3. Keeping your upper body as straight as a plank and breathing out on the way up.

FBI Full Press-up

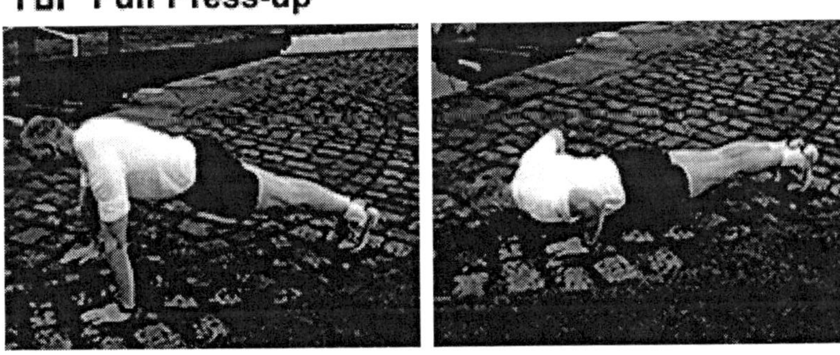

If you're **feeling stronger still:**

1. Adopt a prone position.
2. Keeping the body as straight as a plank with the only points of contact being your hands and your toes.
3. Lower to the floor as one unit keeping straight and as you push back up to the start, breathe out.

Stretching off the worked muscles:

Having worked the Pectorals (chest) and the Triceps (back of your arms), you need to stretch off the muscles accordingly just like we did with the leg muscles after your cardio session. Hold the stretches for about 30 seconds each as shown in the photos.

FBI Triceps Stretch

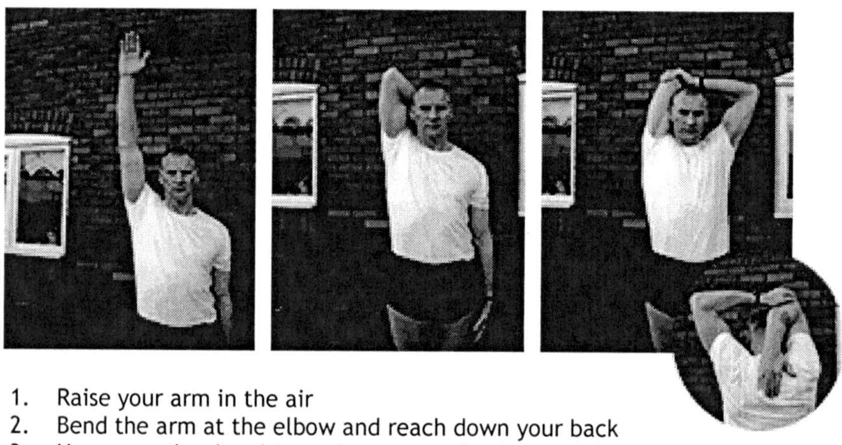

1. Raise your arm in the air
2. Bend the arm at the elbow and reach down your back
3. Use your other hand to push your arm further to obtain a stretch on the back of your arm

FBI Deltoids Stretch

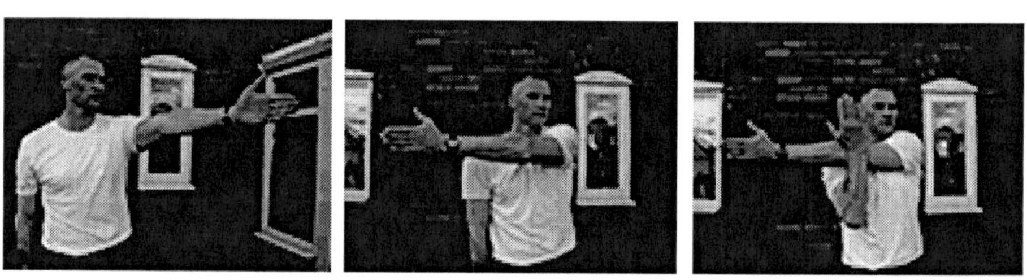

1. Place an arm outstretched in front of you
2. Move it across your body 90 degrees
3. Assist the movement further with your other arm pressing inwards just above your elbow

FBI Pectorals Stretch

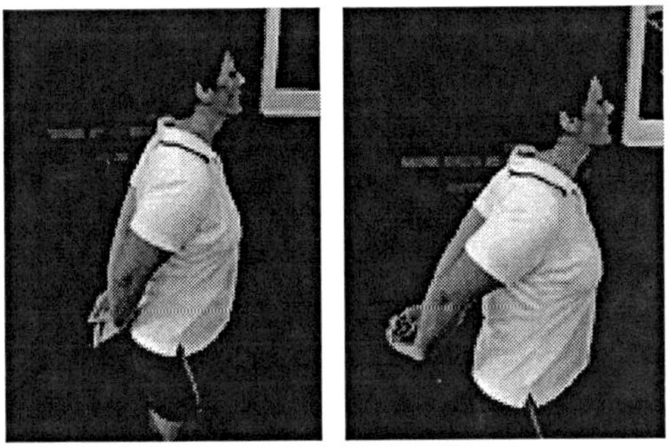

Place your hands behind your back with your palms facing upwards. Move your arms upwards keeping your head upright and push your arms up and away from your body to stretch the muscles of the chest.

FBI Upper Back Stretch

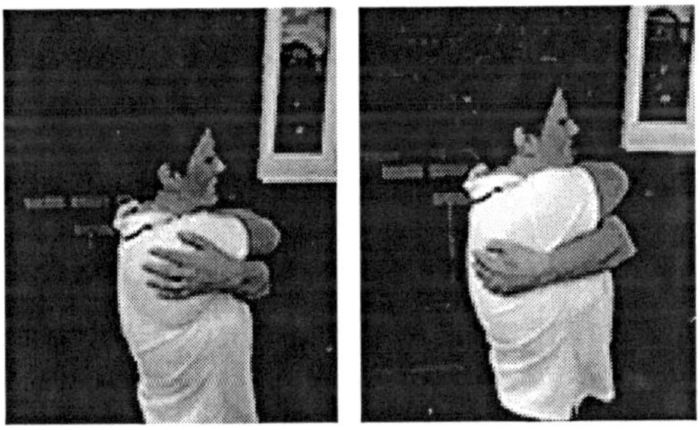

Reach round with both arms as if you're giving yourself a big hug. Breathe in, reach further, hold tight and breathe out. Feel for the stretch in your upper back.

COME ON!

- Do 10 Press-ups starting with the easiest type (the box), moving on to the 3/4 type.
- If you can do 10 of each method move on to the full Press-up.
- Are you still doing the 10 squats every time you sit down? If not, think of the valuable training time that you've already squandered.
- If you are then well done and celebrate with a bonus 20 Squats now!

#14. LEARN TO RELAX

Taking time out to think in silence or maybe playing relaxing music is essential to rid the body of stress.

There are many forms of relaxation techniques out there, try out a few and see which one suits you and your lifestyle. It could be breathing techniques, Yoga, Tai Chi to name but a few.

Carry out some form of relaxation every day. Some people think that a rest day is a wasted day. In training, a planned rest day is necessary and very beneficial. The body needs to recover from a workout so it can repair the muscles and make them stronger.

Prolonged usage without adequate rest will bring on early fatigue and possible injury. It is not essential that you have to rest after every hard session as long as you do build rest days into your program.

Me personally, I do my resting at the weekend, which fits into my routine. Fit your rest days around your normal weekly schedule.

Rest days don't necessarily mean that you can't do anything though. A leisurely walk, cycle or swim etc will do as much for you as a complete rest. Get to know your body and what it responds best to.

COME ON!

- Start to plan out when you are going to exercise and when your rest days will fit in.
- By the time that you have finished the course you will know when it is most suitable for you to train and when you need to put in rest days.
- Relax deeply.

Take a break.

#15. BE PATIENT

Embarking on a total change of life takes time for the body to adapt. But adapt it will, it's what it's good at. Give yourself at least 3 months to notice a change in your body and the way you feel. Other people generally notice the changes in you before you are ready to admit it. You will experience many smaller changes before the 3 months are up but don't expect the earth in a couple of hard weeks. Rest assured though, it will happen.

It is worth remembering how long it took you to get out of condition in the first place. Certain fitness magazines can and will misguide you from time to time and this will really de-motivate you. I have never yet managed to transform an over proportioned belly into a rippling 6 pack in 14 days and I would like to meet the people who have. But over time, these things can be achieved if you work hard at it.

COME ON!

- Reflect on what changes you have made already to your lifestyle.
- Take a glance back at all the tasks that you have been set. Have you done them all?
- Use today's task to catch up on the ones you've let slip.
- If you have done them all, relax back and wallow in your achievement...

#16. FEEL THE CRUNCH

Our next exercise is The Crunch. It is for the abdominal region. If you who are looking for a flat stomach, this is only part of the deal. You must also concentrate on reducing the bodyfat that surrounds the abdominal area by burning those extra calories throughout your day.

Lie down on a suitably cushioned mat. Place your hands behind your head. Raise your knees until your feet are flat on the ground. Keeping your lower back on the floor, breathe out, squeeze your stomach muscles hard and lift your shoulders a couple of inches off the floor. To avoid pulling unnecessarily on your head and neck, push your elbows down towards the ground. Hold the exercise for 5 seconds and return to the floor.

The harder you squeeze, the more your muscles will be working. *Do not hold your breath* in this or any other exercise. If you feel an aching in the neck, it is usual for this exercise until you get used to it. Remember, you are holding your head off the floor, which works the neck muscles. A worked muscle tends to get that aching feeling.

FBI The Crunch

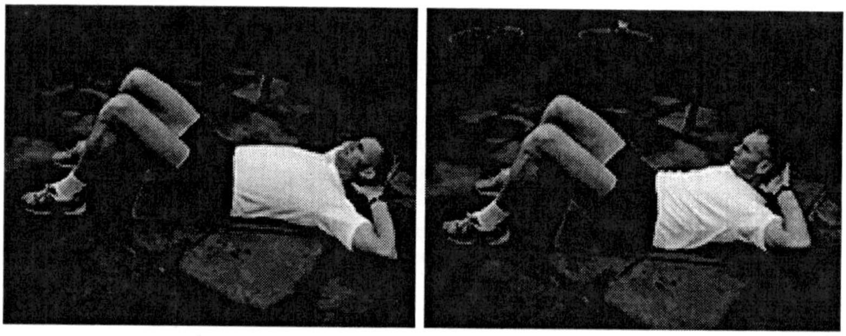

COME ON!

- Carry out 10 Crunches, 10 Press-ups and 10 Squats.
- Rest for 1 minute and repeat.
- This is the building up of your resistance program.

If you're feeling fit then don't feel that you have to stop at the 2 sets, crack on if you can!

#17. KNOW WHY YOU'RE KEEPING FIT

What is your reason for embarking on a new and lasting health and fitness lifestyle?

It may be to lose weight, maintain weight, stave off the effects of a condition (Diabetes, MS etc).

Knowing the reason behind your training and healthy lifestyle will motivate you more. If you are motivated by the physical challenge of one day completing a marathon or by getting into your pre-wedding clothes, always focus on the end result and keep on reminding yourself as to why you are doing this.

You may think that your reasons are selfish. So what? Everyone around you will benefit in one way or another if you are fit and healthy.

COME ON!

- Do your walking/jogging routine.
- If you have not started jogging, just try to jog a small distance followed by a walk.
- This only has to be in short bursts of 10 seconds or the distance between lampposts to start with, building up further each session.

Do it for you!

#18. HAVE A REGULAR MASSAGE

Regular doesn't necessarily mean every week, but you should have a massage at least every couple of months.

Massage has many benefits including, injury prevention, releasing tension in the muscles which can reduce stress levels. Increased permeability of the muscles and skin and you get a definite feel good factor. Any one of those reasons alone is a good enough excuse for a massage, so grouped together you can see why I place such value on them.

There are different types of massage from the all body relaxing "Swedish Massage" to the more specific and vigorous deep tissue "Sports Massage". Depending on your particular needs at that time, there is no better way to treat your body than to lie back and let someone else move your muscles for you for a change.

I tend to treat many clients for muscle injuries caused by over exertion of an inflexible or weak muscle. Remember that prevention is better than cure.

COME ON!

- Find out the reputable therapists in your area.
- Find out what kind of massage or treatments they specialise in.
- It's always good to know where you can go for treatments in advance.

You and your body deserve it - so treat yourself

#19. LEARNING THE ROPES

Today we will look at a different cardio session. All you need is a piece of rope and enough room to swing a cat (not literally). If you did skipping at school, you will reminisce of hours and hours of skipping in the playground. You will soon see how fit you must have been back then because it can be quite taxing. Skipping requires good co-ordination as well as stamina and endurance.

I prefer to use what is called a “speed rope”, which you can get from most sports outlets. It is the closest thing to the old washing lines. Careful though, it doesn’t half smart when you snag. If you’ve never skipped since school or not at all then you’re in for some serious fun. The worse you are at first the more energy you will expend so there’s an excellent trade off. The body and mind will soon realise just how high you’re jumping in relation to the thickness of the rope and will bring you closer to the ground each time you skip.

Skip two-footed landing lightly on the balls of your feet. I tend to use skipping as a warm-up exercise as well as a cardio session. A few minutes skipping will soon bring your heart rate up to a good working level. If you’re thinking of going into the boxing world, then let me introduce you to your everlasting training companion... The Rope

COME ON!

- Cardio Session time.
- Skip for 1 minute with 30 seconds rest.
- Repeat until you have done 10 sets.
- Record how many skips you do for each minute and see the overall improvement each time you carry out a session.
- If you do not have a rope at this stage, then get out and pace the pavement and remember to record your distance.

#20. ENJOY YOUR FOOD

Food is essential to the body so enjoy the pleasure of eating. If you exercise regularly and eat the right foods, you will be able to eat extremely well. Probably more than you've ever done before if you are one of the "Diet" brigade.

Eat your food nice and slow. The slower that you eat your food, the more satisfying it is. Not much in life beats a leisurely meal in good company. Chew all your food well to assist digestion. Take time out for eating, plan it into your day and try not to eat on the hoof.

If you are one of the millions who say that you don't have time to eat, consider this. I bet you always find time in your day to fill up the car with fuel if you're going on a journey. Why? Because you will have already built in that time into your schedule. Do the same for your precious body.

COME ON!

- Take a break for meals - at least half an hour to eat leisurely.
- Enjoy the experience.
- Build this in to your daily routine for the future.

Get that good fuel down your neck.

#21. LATERAL THINKING

Today's exercise is the Lateral Raise. Lateral meaning sideways. This exercise will develop the Deltoid muscle group in the shoulders. You need dumbbells or similar objects for both hands. You could use a couple of tins of beans or even full water bottles etc.

Stand with your knees slightly bent (soft knees) and a neutral spine (natural hollow in the back). With the weights at your side, lift them out to the side so the arms are parallel to the floor. Maintain the same angle at the elbow throughout the movement. Slightly rotate the wrists forward (as if pouring from a jug) as you get to the top of the movement. Breathe out on the way up. Return your hands to your side under control and that is one repetition.

FBI **Lateral Raises**

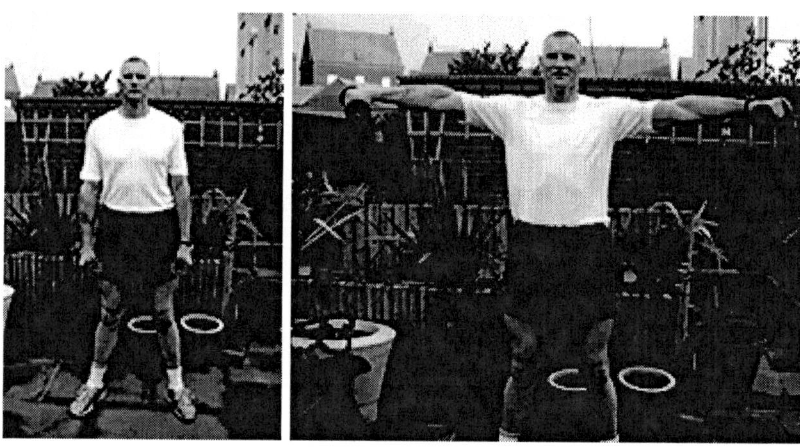

COME ON!

- 10 Squats - 10 Press-ups - 10 Crunches - 10 Lateral Raises.
- 1 minute rest and repeat the sequence.

Always make sure that you keep to the strictest form when you are exercising.

#22. REFUEL AFTER A WORKOUT

Ideally, after a hard training session, you should refuel as soon as possible. This is more important if you're thinking of becoming a serious athlete where good nutrition is absolutely essential.

We will first look at what an athlete should consume then tinker it to suit a non-athlete.

The most effective way to refuel after training is to consume carbohydrates. To obtain the carbohydrate needed, you need to eat 50 grams of carbohydrate immediately following training, then a further 50 grams every 30 minutes up to the end of 2 hours. This will result in 250 grams being consumed during these 2 hours. This will prevent the athlete feeling "phased" by a large meal immediately following training, as well as maximising digestion and absorption.

If the athlete ultimately cannot consume solids immediately following training, then an isotonic sports drink will suffice.

The meal following this carbohydrate replenishment phase should consist of both protein and carbohydrate. Meat or fish with potatoes, rice or pasta is a good combination.

So where does that leave the not so serious athlete who has other things to do other than time their meals? We can still consume a carbohydrate snack straight after a workout. A Banana sandwich (2 slices) is ideal. An isotonic drink would also suffice. Basically there are many easy to prepare foods that you could get your required carbs within 2 hours of your workout. Cereals, vegetable soup, jacket spud (baked potato) with a low fat filling. So we don't have to be too different from the professionals do we?

COME ON!

- Cardio Session time.
- Skipping for 1 minute with 30 seconds rest.
- Repeat until you have done 10 sets.

- Record how many skips you do for each minute and see if you can improve on the last time you did this.
- If you still do not have a rope, it's another run/jog for you.

If you want to add some variety to your cardio, go on, buy a rope!

#23. BUILD YOUR OWN TRAINING PROGRAM

Today we are going to look at starting to build a training program with the exercises that we already know.

This can obviously be added to as we learn new exercises, building up into a comprehensive program to substantially change your body shape (if that is what you are after). You can use the template provided or make up your own. The content is more important than the layout.

The training program is split into two main parts. The cardio section and the resistance section.

I have not included the actions of the warm-up or cool-down with stretches as this remains the same and should always be a part of the whole session. So it only gets a mention in title only. The exercises can be done in pen but do the weights and reps in pencil as they will change throughout the course. A more permanent training program can be devised at the end of the course, as you will have the knowledge to tweak the program to match your aim.

There's a blank Exercise Program Sheet for you to use on the next page which you can also download and print out for free here: www.stevehalls.com/fbi-charts

Under the "weight" section, we are using body (which is our own bodyweight) for most of the exercises at the moment. This will change as you get more proficient and stronger.

To establish the work rate we use sets/reps. for example 2 x 10 is equal to 2 sets of 10 exercises with a rest in between. The rest period we are using at the moment is 30 seconds.

EXERCISE PROGRAM SHEET

EXERCISE	DURATION	REMARKS
Warm-up	10 mins	Your mobilising and warm-up routine

EXERCISE	SETS/REPS	WEIGHT	REMARKS
COOLDOWN AND STRETCH			

COME ON!

- Copy the template from the previous page or go online www.stevehalls.com/fbi-charts and print it off and start to fill out your program.
- Get to know what all the boxes are used for.
- We will be filling this in with more exercises as we travel on our fitness journey.

We'll catch up again tomorrow.

#24. BREAKFAST LIKE A KING

Start the day with a substantial breakfast.

You saw what I have on most days when we started the food diary on day 8.

Light the calorie burning ovens within your lean muscle mass early in the day. You would fill up your car with petrol before a long journey, so do the same to your body. This raises the metabolism, which will help you to burn more calories throughout the day.

We wake up with a low blood sugar level so it is important to get the levels up as soon as possible. If you skip breakfast your body will in effect be lying dormant until that first feed. If that first feed is not till lunchtime or beyond, just think of the time you've wasted not burning calories.

Start the day with a nice slow burning carbohydrate like porridge, cereals or wholemeal toast etc. Pasta is a great source too, but many would not consider eating this for breakfast.

COME ON!

- Start your day with a substantial breakfast.
- Build in the time for a good breakfast before you leave for work.
- You may have to get up a bit earlier, but it is the "early bird that catches the worm" remember.

See the difference this makes to your day.

#25. THE UPRIGHT ROW

Today's new exercise is the Upright Row. This uses two major muscles in this exercise. Your Trapezium, which is the muscle that lies across the back of your shoulders up to your neck. Plus your Biceps, which are the muscles on the front of your upper arms. Using your resistance weights, stand with the weights in front of you, resting on your thighs. Leading with your elbows, lift the weights up to the top of your chest breathing out as you lift. Return the weights to the bottom under control. Ensure that the weights stay close to the body throughout the movement. Keep a timing of 2 seconds for the up movement and 2 seconds for the down.

FBI Upright Row

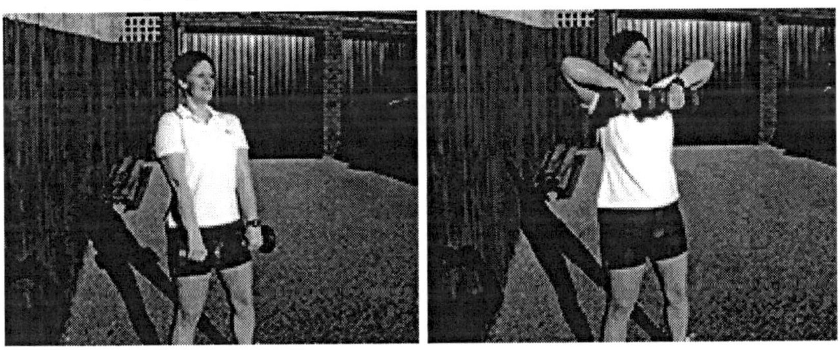

COME ON!

- Add Upright Row 2 sets of 10 reps (2 x 10) with Dumbbells to your training program and carry out the resistance exercises.
- Always make sure that you keep to the strictest form when you are exercising.
- Tomorrow we'll look at working outside your comfort zone and explain it fully.

Prepare to go to another level!

#26. THE COMFORT ZONE AND BEYOND

I've mentioned your comfort zone a few times already in this course so it's time I talked about it further. For the body to make changes, you need to do something that it struggles to do. For example, if you can easily do 10 press-ups or run a mile. Then just doing that time after time will not give you the changes in body composition (bodyfat/lean muscle) that you're seeking. In that instance you would be working within your comfort zone.

So how do you know when you are stepping out of this comfort zone? Well, you must first know what it means to run or do cardio-vascular exercise at what is termed "Comfortable Pace". There are a few signs to look out for that will tell you. These are:

- Your breathing changes from Nose Breathing to Mouth Breathing.
- If talking, you need to pick your moment to speak in short sentences. On that, one word at a time is too fast and long paragraphs means you're going too slowly.
- If you're using a heart rate monitor (I'll speak more about training with one of these later on in the course) you should be about 70% of your maximum heart rate if you're already fit. Don't worry about this too much now, it will all become quite clear.
- You should feel as if you can go on for much longer at this or at a slower pace. This can be from 5 minutes for a de-conditioned person to 2 hours plus for an elite athlete.
- Your facial expression should be such that you know you are exercising, but are not experiencing discomfort.

Now we know what it means to be training at "Comfortable Pace", we will therefore know what to do to take it beyond this to start to tax the body.

Remember, that if you do what you've always done, you'll always get what you've always got. So to make changes we must do something that the body finds taxing and difficult.

In running etc it's trying to beat your best times, distance etc.

In resistance training it's trying to work your muscles until they are fatigued and therefore have to stop. If you can now do 10 press-ups, "up the ante", go for 20. Aim high. This goes for all resistance exercises. I will tell you how to include this into your training program very soon.

COME ON!

- Carry out your full cardio routine
- Mobility
- Warm-up
- Run or Skip, out of your comfort zone
- Cool down and stretch

Now record your time? Will it be better? It should be.

#27. FRESH IS BEST

It is always much better eating food straight from where your creator (who-ever you believe in) intended.

Fresh food is nutritionally better than something that comes out of a packet or tin.

If you think of a line of food with fresh organic food at one end and "Fast Food" at the other; all foods belong somewhere on that line.

We are in control of the fresh food that we cook but if we take our daily calories from fast food, we are at the mercy of the food outlets by not knowing exactly what they have done with it. This is how my line looks. Best first of course.

Home Grown	Fresh Organic	Fresh	Frozen	Tin/Packet/Jar	Fast Food
BEST					WORST

Depending on the ingredients of the processed foods will depend whether or not I promote them or relegate them down the list.

Processed food that is put in a can, jar or packet usually comes with a host of additives and "E" numbers which the body does not need.

Half the additives you won't even be able to pronounce, so why eat them. Your body has only got to get rid of them. So just save your body the unnecessary work by not taking them in.

Processed food also generally contains a fair amount of added sugar, salt or fat to make it taste better.

COME ON!

- Today is a rest day from exercise.
- Have a look in your cupboards and check out some of those labels.
- Can you pronounce all the ingredients in a relatively simple product?
- How much fresh food do you have in today? Is there any improvement that you can address the next time you go shopping? If so, do it.

Remember, fresh is best.

#28. LUNCH LIKE A PRINCE

So you've begun to breakfast like a king, so what about lunchtime?

A healthy lunch will top up that engine and keep you moving throughout the day. Slow releasing carbohydrate ensures that we don't get a sudden "sugar spike" and the fall in blood sugar that follows. Pasta, jacket potatoes with a low fat filling, chicken salad, wholemeal bread with a homemade vegetable soup are examples of simple but healthy lunches.

Don't overeat if your "main meal" is normally later in the day, but ensure that you do have enough to get you through the afternoon without reaching for the unhealthy snack. It is when you leave yourself hungry that temptation rears its ugly head. The reason for this is quite straightforward. The brain is fed by fresh glucose from the bloodstream. The glucose in your bloodstream is broken down carbohydrate. When your blood sugar level falls, the brain calls out for glucose. The snag is that it wants it quick, so a healthy starchy food, which is recommended, will not satisfy the brain. Enter the chocolate biscuit etc. Full of simple sugars which can be broken down by the digestive enzymes quickly. They enter the bloodstream quickly and there goes your "sugar spike" once more.

Back to the car journey... Don't we usually top up the tank again along the way? Or are you a risky sort who leaves it to the last minute and drives into a strange city running on nothing but fumes? Feel the confidence of not running out of fuel in the afternoon, have your healthy lunch like a prince.

COME ON!

- It's time for the full cardio program again.
- Skipping yet? Come on make more of an effort if you haven't started.
- Remember, variety is the spice of life.

Keep recording those times. Plot a graph to show you how much progress you are making.

#29. BROAD SHOULDERS

Today's exercise is the Shoulder Press.

It can be performed standing or sitting down it doesn't really matter.

The important thing is the action of the working muscles, the "Deltoids" which are the main shoulder muscles and the "Triceps", which are on the back of your upper arms.

Holding your weights in front of your body under your chin with your palms facing towards you. Raise both your hands until fully extended putting in a half twist of the wrists so that your palms now face away from your body.

Breathe out on the way up. Count for 2 seconds on the way up, hold the weights steady and count to two on the way down again.

That's it, simple as that. Points to note are:

1. Keep the spine neutral - don't arch it to try and lift heavier weights than you're capable of.
2. Keep your knees soft throughout the exercise if you're standing up.

FBI Shoulder Press

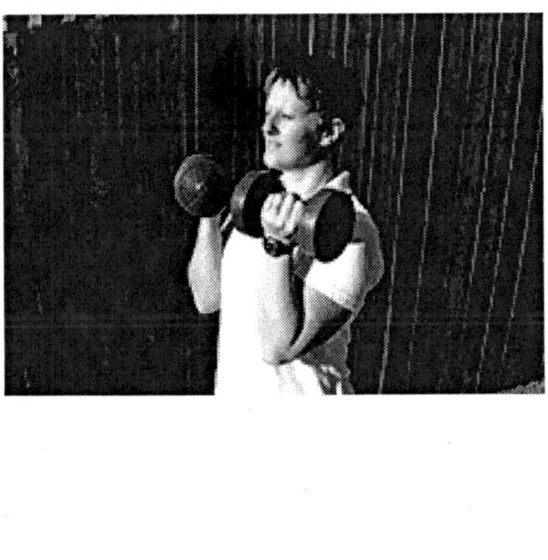

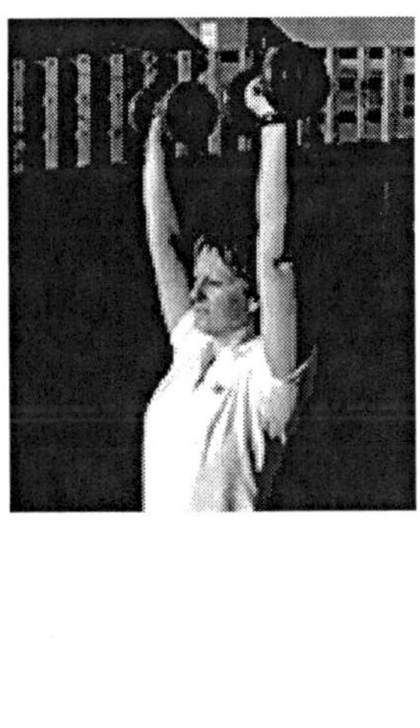

COME ON!

- Add the shoulder Press to your training program 2 x 10 with weights
- Change your Press-ups from 2 x 10 to 2 x fatigue.
- This means do as many as you can, rest, then do them again.
- Start to use your weights when carrying out the squats.

Alter your program accordingly. Glad you used your pencil now?

#30. MAKE A LIST – STICK TO THE LIST

Go food shopping with a plan. This sounds so obvious, most good advice *is* plainly obvious, but it doesn't stop us mere mortals from missing it from time to time.

Always remember, if it's not in the cupboards you can't eat it so you have to be strong and resolute once and that's when you go food shopping.

Only buy what you need, not what you fancy at the time.

Plan for the week ahead with a healthy nutritional menu. Work out what you need for the week using as much fresh produce as possible and go prepared. This also saves money. Be careful with special offers. We all like to get a bargain but sometimes it makes us buy something for the sake of it.

"Buy one get one free" or similar offers on a packet of biscuits might tempt you to buy something that wasn't on your list because it was an offer your purse (or wallet) couldn't refuse. Save even more money - don't buy the original product.

Never go shopping when you're hungry. This is a disaster waiting to happen. Your trolley will end up with all sorts of goodies (or is that baddies?) that you did not intend to buy when you first went shopping. The smell of food starts your digestive juices flowing, that's what the body does. Your mouth waters, getting ready to break down the food that it craves and is getting ready for. However, when your stomach is full of nutritionally good fuel the brain is being fed with fresh glucose steadily and you don't get the same response.

Buy what you intend to eat not eat what you buy.

COME ON!

- A rest day from exercise.
- Make your shopping list for the following week.
- If you include tins, packets or jars, see if you could change that for a fresh alternative.

Stick to the list. Because if it's not in the cupboards you can't eat it!

#31. PAIN OR DISCOMFORT?

Ever heard someone say, I don't do that exercise, it hurts my back? I have many, many times.

Some of those people avoid working the muscle to such a degree that there is muscle wastage in that area. This means that when you try and exercise that body part, you get pain and soreness. It is an ever-decreasing circle that needs to be broken.

A weak back needs to be made strong so you have to know the difference between what is pain and what is discomfort due to exercise. If you lift a "light weight", which you find relatively easy and you get a sharp twinge or stabbing pain in a localised area, then that is pain. This is your body telling you that something is wrong. If you ignore this and work through it you are doing yourself no good whatsoever. This is the time to see a Sports Therapist or your GP and get some remedial treatment.

If you get a fatigued feeling after constant repetition through a build up of lactic acid, the pain and difficulty seems to increase with each repetition, then this is discomfort. This is acceptable to the body as you are clearly working outside your comfort zone which will make your body adapt i.e. change. If you persevere with the exercise the discomfort decreases with each workout. Beware though it could reoccur when you "up" the intensity or duration. You might have already experienced that earlier in the course.

COME ON!

- Has it really been a month already?
- How much has your running improved?
- If you started out walking or jogging, are you up to the next level?
- If the answer to the last 2 questions is "yes" then be impressed, I am.
- It's time to increase the cardio session by 5 minutes.

Build the time into your program and go to it champ!

#32. TAKE THE P'LUNGE

Today we are introducing another leg exercise for our resistance program. This is called the Lunge. This exercise works the upper thighs and bum in general but it also helps you to balance.

FBI The Lunge

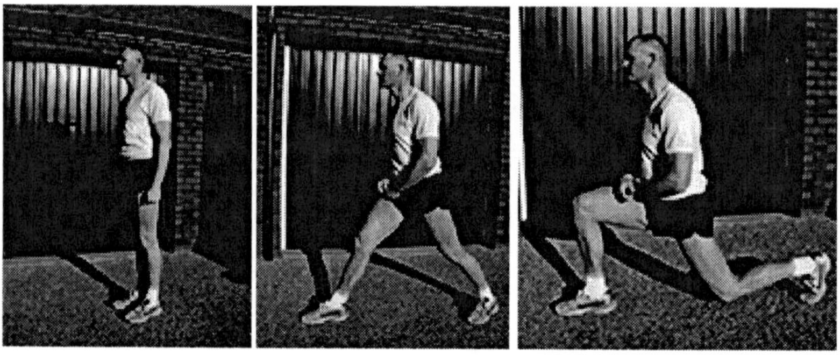

- **Stage 1:** Stand with your legs and your feet together.
- **Stage 2:** Take an extended pace forward keeping your feet straight.
- **Stage 3:** Lower your rear knee to the floor. Don't bang it on the floor it really hurts, I know. The front knee should not go forward of your toes. The control comes from the rear leg. It is this one that you will really feel working.
- **Stage 4:** Raise your rear knee so you are at the extended pace position again as in stage 2.
- **Repeat stages 3 and 4** for as many times as the training program dictates.
- **Stage 5:** Bring your front foot back in line with your rear foot.
- **Repeat** the procedure changing the working leg.

Always look straight ahead and keep your body upright. This does take a bit of practice. If at first your balance seems hopeless don't worry there are tips to help you to get more proficient. Stand very close to a wall or something that is comfortable to lean on. If you lose your balance, you will just lean but not fall over. Gradually, you will get to the point where you won't need any props to assist you. The more tired your legs become in the exercise, the harder you will have to work to maintain your balance. Stick with it, you will improve, trust me.

COME ON!

- Add Lunges to the training program.
- Start with 5 on each leg with a 1 minute rest, followed by a second set.

Come on, take the P'lunge.

#33. CRUISE WITH THE BOOZE

Ever been on a "Booze Cruise"? The aim is normally to drink as much as you can within the given trip time.

If you have done that, (like me in my earlier days I must confess), change your mind set and "Cruise with the Booze".

1g of alcohol = 7 calories. It's easy to consume many calories through alcohol. Alcohol in large amounts is also toxic to the body. Therefore your body has to rid itself of this before it causes permanent damage.

This puts a strain on the liver and kidneys to cleanse the blood. If these organs are working "full-on" with this task, then it stands to reason that they are not performing their normal function to the same capability.

You can liken this to a workforce who has enough manpower to do a set number of tasks in a given time frame. You increase the load without increasing the manpower or time frame and what do you get? A job that may not be done to the best standards or you end up with a very tired worn out workforce.

A lot of alcohol has other implications in the health and fitness world. I don't know many (if any) people who train as good and hard as they normally do after a good "skin full". Do you? It also tends to put you off guard in the healthy diet world - e.g. 10 pints and a curry etc. I think most of us have been there at one time or another.

Now the beauty of this 90-day course is it's sustainable and sensible. So I'm not for one moment saying that you should not have a drink, but I am saying that drink is calories, it is toxic in large quantities and it does incapacitate to a degree. Drink sensibly and enjoy both worlds.

COME ON!

- Have a relax.
- Mull over the past few days and see if there are any outstanding tasks that you should have done.
- Bet you thought I was going to tell you to have a drink.
- Never, that's always your decision nobody else's.

Take it easy.

#34. LIMIT THE SALT

Do you remember I mentioned yesterday about the danger of your organs working overtime due to too much alcohol? Well the same applies when we eat too much salt in our diet.

For every gram of salt consumed, the body is said to retain 70g of water. The kidneys retain water to dilute the salt and this overloading of the kidneys can lead to high blood pressure and strokes, coronary heart disease and kidney failure. The chemical name for salt is Sodium Chloride. It is the Sodium that is potentially harmful. Sodium can appear in other substances used in food manufacture.

For example:

- Sodium Citrate
- Sodium Bicarbonate - Baking Powder
- Sodium Sulphate - to bleach fruit
- Sodium Benzoate - in salad dressings and chutneys
- Sodium Ascorbate - added to vitamin tablets
- Monosodium Glutamate (MSG)
- Brine

We usually take in 95% of our sodium from salt and so we usually talk about salt intake rather than sodium intake. For the body to process the salt it must retain water. Water retention can lead to weight increase and higher blood pressure. There is generally enough natural salt in the foods we eat without adding to it.

There are 4 main sources of sodium in our diet:

- The salt pot at the table
- Salt added during cooking
- Salt added in food processing
- Natural salt in foods

We only need about 2g of salt daily. This should ideally come from a good "wholefood" diet and therefore there is no need to have any additional salt.

Seafoods are the main foods that are naturally high in salt. Kidneys are a good source and so are vegetables such as celery and chicory.

A lot of people add salt to their food without even tasting the food first. What an insult to the chef that is! Would you like to slave over a stove and see your creation covered in ketchup or other sauces? Probably not, so why do it with salt?

Simple strategies to cut down on salt:

- Remove the salt pot from the table
- Taste the food first
- Use more herbs and spices to enhance the flavour of foods during cooking
- In cooking, gradually reduce the amount you use

COME ON!

- Use the simple strategies to start to reduce your salt intake.
- Cardio session today. Let's get out and break some records.
- Record your results.

Cut down on that salt, it's important

#35. V FOR VICTORY

Today we are going to add another abdominal exercise to the resistance routine. The new exercise is called a "Vee Sit". You need your mat or a suitably cushioned floor for this exercise.

FBI Vee Sit

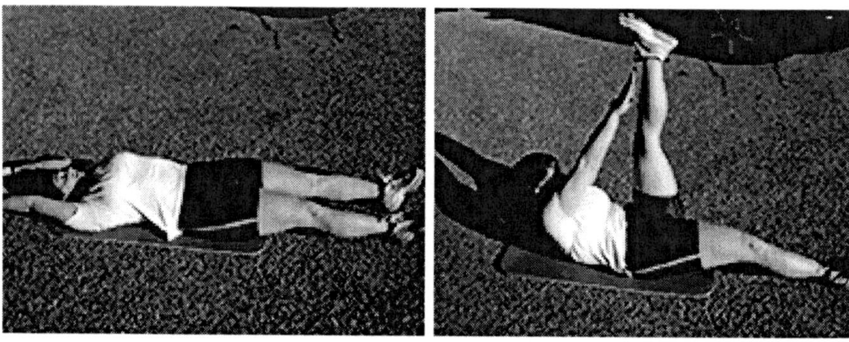

Lie down flat on the floor and raise your arms above your head. Keeping your leg straight raise it in the air until you reach 90 degrees of travel. So it should by now be straight up in the air. Simultaneously, raise your torso bringing your raised arms past your head until you touch your shin. Lower back down to the starting position and repeat the action with the opposite leg.

When you have perfected this exercise you can make it harder by a simple adjustment to the action. When your hands touch your shins, reach up and try to touch your feet. The higher you reach, the harder the exercise. Make sure you keep your leg straight though.

COME ON!

- Add this exercise to the routine.
- Put in 2 x 10 (5 on each leg)

Tomorrow, we will review your training program so far.

#36. TRAINING PROGRAM REVIEW

As we have added a few exercises to the training program since we started, I thought we would just take a look at what it should look like if you are using the template provided in lesson 23. This is really to confirm that we are still on the same wavelength.

If you are using your own design, it should have all the relevant information.

This is what my program looks like so far...

EXERCISE	DURATION	REMARKS	
Warm-up	10 mins	Your mobilising and warm-up routine	
Walk/Jog/Run	25 mins	Try to beat your previous distance. When 12.5 minutes out turn round and head home.	
Skipping	20 mins	14 intervals of 1 minute rounds. 30 seconds rest. Record the amount per minute (seek progress)	
EXERCISE	**SETS/REPS**	**WEIGHT**	**REMARKS**
Pressups	2 x fatigue	Body	Keep your body straight.
Squats	2 x 10	Dumbells	Knees not forward of toes.
Crunches	2 x 10	Body	Squeeze stomach muscles. Hold for 5 seconds.
Lateral Raise	2 x 10	Dumbells	Twist the wrists forwards.
Upright Row	2 x 10	Dumbells	Lead with your elbows.
Shoulder Press	2 x 10	Dumbells	Twist the wrists as you lift.
Lunges	2 x 10	Body	Rear leg controls the movement. 5 on each leg.
Vee Sits	2 x 10	Body	Keep legs straight. 5 on each leg.
COOLDOWN AND STRETCH			

I've got dumbbells as the weights, but you can use anything that is balanced. Water bottles, milk cartons, bricks etc.

As we are building up the resistance program, it is inevitable that the time for completion is getting longer and longer. It is reasonable to have a training session last for one hour. If however you are finding that time is getting tight, you can always split the exercises into two days. If you do this, make sure you do complete all the exercises so that your body remains in balance. Men have a tendency to overdo their chests if anything. It is better at this stage though to keep making time to do the routine.

COME ON!

- Take a rest day from exercise.
- Update your training program if it differs radically from mine.

Keep it up!

#37. EAT FRESH PRODUCE – IN SEASON

When choosing fresh fruit or vegetables, pick the varieties that are in season. These taste far better than "forced" varieties. A lot of what you buy is out of your sphere of influence especially in the case of exotic type fruit and vegetables that are not from your native country.

Farm shops are good sources for these products. Organically produced food is normally a better option if maybe a little more expensive. Buying direct from the farmers is usually cheaper so look out for the "Fresh Produce" signs that spring up over the year. At least you know that it is as fresh as it can be. Food is meant to be enjoyable and fresher food tastes better.

If possible grow your own and see the difference in taste between your variety and the shop bought one. You will be amazed. A bit of digging is also a good cardio exercise, but I won't include it in your program.

COME ON!

- Cardio session again.
- Hands up if you are still not skipping.
- But, if you are still making progress, I will let you off.

Fresh is best, when it's in season it's better!

#38. "PUT YOUR BACK INTO IT"

Today we are going to add a lower back exercise to the program. This is called a "Dorsal Raise".

It is very important to train all the muscles to get an even balance to the body, but the lower back is often ignored. Often, it is ignored because of a perceived "bad back".

A weak back needs strengthening. If you do not train the back it becomes weak and you get muscle wastage in that area. Subsequently when you try to work the back it hurts. So what is the way round it? Do back exercises regularly, especially if you've worked your abdominal muscles. Be careful though, remember day 31, pain or discomfort?

If you need to refresh do that before you carry out the exercise. If it does hurt I would get yourself off to a Sports Therapist for a consultation and treatment. If your back is weak now and you do nothing about it, it will only get weaker through time and give you more trouble in your later years.

So, to the exercise:

FBI Dorsal Raise

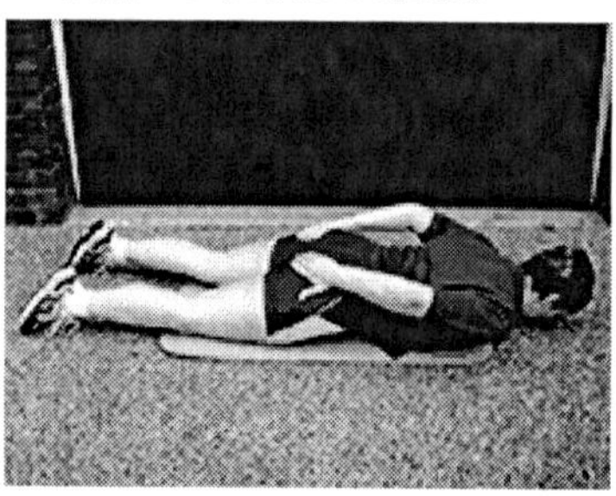

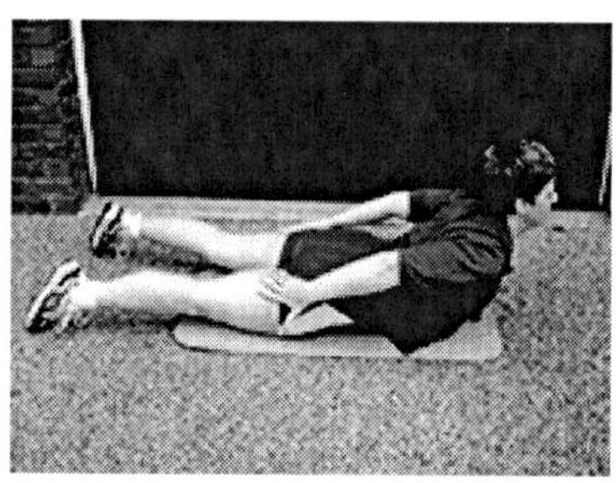

1. Lie down on your front with your hands behind your back.
2. Keep your feet on the ground at all times.
3. Raise your shoulders off the ground and hold it for 5 seconds.
4. Whilst you're raising, push your hands as far down the backs of your thighs as you can.
5. Breathe out slowly as you perform the movement.
6. Return to the start position ready for another rep.

You should feel the muscles in the lower back as you lift. If you can't at this stage don't worry. "If you're lifting you're working". For most people there is not a lot of movement involved in this exercise, me especially. It all depends on the flexibility of the spine. It will improve though, so work it through your natural range of motion and work it hard.

For progression, you can do the variants as shown in the photos. a) shows the hands underneath the chin. Progressing further to b) where your arms are outstretched to the side and the final progression is with your arms outstretched to the front like c).

Remember to perfect your exercise before moving on to the next level.

FBI Dorsal Raise (variations)

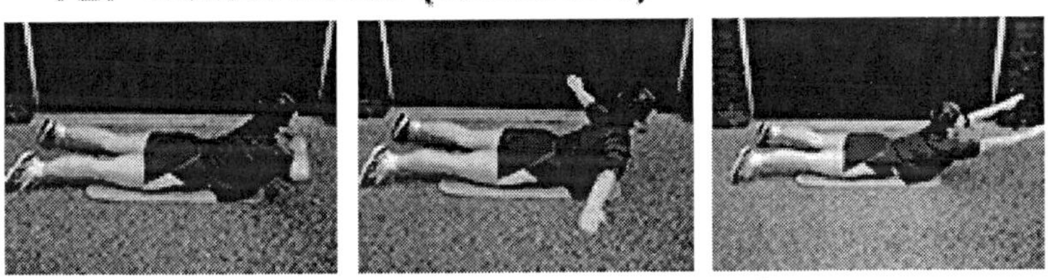

a) b) c)

COME ON!

- Add the "Dorsal Raise" to your routine and perform 2 sets of 10 reps - 2 x 10
- And remember to "put your back into it".

#39. DO NOT UNDER-EAT OR STARVE YOURSELF

Be careful that in your efforts to cut down on some of your food intake, that you don't under eat. This is as bad as overeating, some say worse because there are not the nutrients going into the body that it needs for everyday functions.

Your body will close down if you starve it. It will also hold on to bodyfat in a bid to "survive the famine". Your body will use your proteins (muscle, hormones etc) as fuel. This will lead to a reduced amount of lean muscle in the body, which burns your calories.

So having spent over a month trying to build up your lean muscle, you would be using it up as fuel at the same time. Now, what a waste of time that would be.

If this is the case, when you start eating again you subsequently have less muscle to utilise the energy, which in turn means that there is fuel unused in the body. This is absorbed and stored in the body as bodyfat. The loss of weight on the scales is generally down to less muscle and therefore less water in the body.

Have you ever wondered why all these people, and you might be included in this, get fatter after a diet? Enter the "Yo-Yo". We've all heard about yo-yo dieters, well this is why they get it wrong.

So no more will you starve, or crave food night and day, because as you know now, we feed our body the nutrients that it desires.

We will talk later in the course about specifics like weight loss and muscle building, but for now just feed and be healthy, you might already be losing weight as I write.

COME ON!

- Let us re-visit your food diary.
- Have you been keeping it up? Remember, you cannot change what you don't know.
- If you stick to much the same foods week after week it becomes very easy.
- Are you taking in the right amount of food and water? If not, now is the time to change it. If you are "well done" you're a star.

Remember - eat what you need.

#40. EAT A RAINBOW

One of the best ways to eat a balanced diet is to "Eat a Rainbow". It is a simple statement that means so much.

We know that "variety is the spice of life", well in nutrition, it's no different. Different coloured foods have differing vitamins and minerals. Take fruit for example, for your daily portions, instead of 4 or 5 apples, wouldn't it be better to see an array of colours such as Red Apple, Oranges, Yellow Banana, Green Kiwi, Blueberries. That is just a start.

Vegetables are the same. If you look down at your meal and see just one colour, how appetising does it look? Again, try and get different colours on your plate. People generally eat with their eyes first, if it looks awful, are you really going to want it? Probably not. Why do you think food manufactures spend so much time putting in artificial colouring into foods? Yes, you've guessed it, to make us buy it.

Today in our cardio section, I'm going to show you an easy to perform exercise using a box. It is called a "Straddle Jump":

1. Stand by the side of your box with your nearest foot on top of the box (first photo).
2. Ensure that the box is steady and will not move under the weight of you jumping on it.
3. Push downwards with your foot that's on the box and lift your other leg off the floor.
4. Place that foot also on the box next to your first foot (second photo).
5. Shift your weight to the other side of the box and lower your first foot to the floor (third photo).

You can make this harder by jumping from one side to the other having only one foot on the box at a time. By increasing the height of the box or increasing the speed of the exercise, you can increase the intensity of the exercise.

FBI Straddle Jump

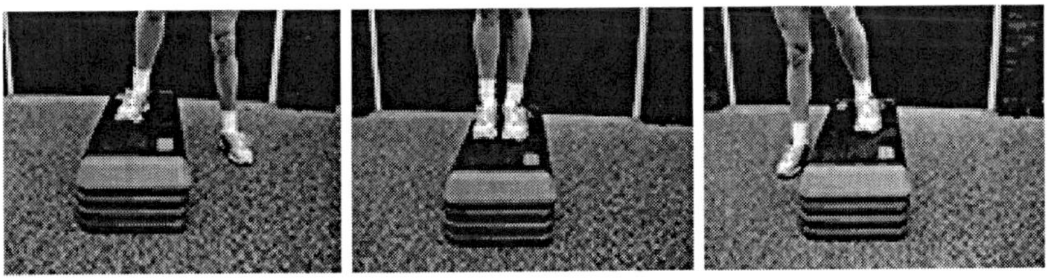

A suggested time frame for the straddle jumps would be 30 seconds work with 1-minute rest for starters. Build this up so you are doing 1-minute work and 30 seconds rest. Always look for improvement in the same way that you do with your running and skipping.

COME ON!

- Cardio day today
- Pick any one of 3 or make a routine of your own.
- Remember, it is your program. You control it and not the other way round.

Add this new exercise to your program and go for it.

#41. ARE YOU A BIT "DIPPY"?

Well believe it or not, you're going to be.

Today's resistance exercise is the "Tricep Dip".

This exercise is for the back of your arm, the muscle group called the "Triceps". For ladies in the UK, it gets rid of the potential "Bingo Wings". I'm not sure what other names people use throughout the world, although I'll probably find out very soon.

It's a simple exercise that can be performed as you sit now on your chair at your computer screen. If you're brave enough that is.

FBI Tricep Dip

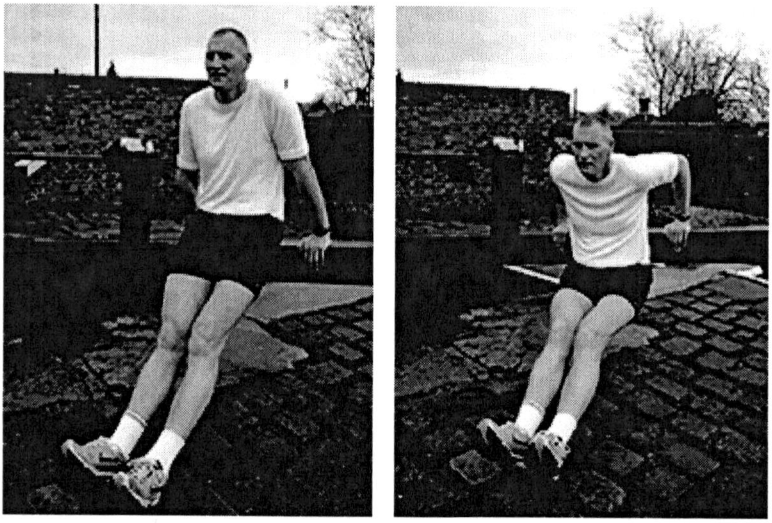

1. Use a bench, chair or as my picture suggests, a canal lock. Have a sit down (very temporarily).
2. Place your hands on the bench at your side shoulder width apart.
3. Lower your body until your elbows are at an angle of 90 degrees.
4. Push back up so the body returns to the starting position, breathing out on the way up.

5. Ensure that your back remains close to the bench throughout the movement.

There you have it, so you may be dippy after all.

COME ON!

- Add the "Tricep Dips" to your training program 2 x 10.
- Carry out your full resistance training routine.

I hope you warm up, cool down and stretch properly. Remember, it is all part of the full package, always carry out the basics. Build in the time required.

#42. RESPECT NIGGLES

Little niggles turn into proper injuries when left untreated.

Now that you are getting fitter and taking the time to live a healthy life it is important to stay injury free.

Injuries lead to unforced rest periods in your training and may even affect your work. If you're self-employed, like me, you know how much this has to be avoided. No work = No money.

Listen to your body, if it hurts then stop the activity and train something else or train in a different way so there is no pain. I always say that an injury is an opportunity to train another body part. It's never an excuse for stopping all your activities. Does that ring a bell from your past?

Masking the pain with painkilling substances only delay the unwanted outcome. Using heat treatments either hot or cold mask your injury in the following way. In "layman's" terms heat signals from the body to the brain arrive quicker than the pain signals. Therefore the brain does not register the pain only the heat.

Did your Mother ever rub your arm fast and vigorously when you knocked it? More still, did it soothe you? The answer is probably yes in both instances. Your Mother and her Mother before her knew more than they thought about anatomy and physiology. But remember, you are still injured and are likely to be making it much worse if you ignore the signs.

COME ON!

- A rest day and a chance to catch up on the few items that you may have let slip.

Stick with it, you're doing great!

#43. QUALITY OVER QUANTITY

For years people have been saying that in order to lose weight you need to cut down on your food. The focus therefore is usually on the quantity. Whilst it is true that quantity does play a part, I find that quality plays a much bigger part.

How many people have you known who have tried to cut down in a bid to lose weight? You might even be one of them. More to the point, who do you know who has tried it more than once? Quite simply, it's madness to do the same thing over and over again and expect different results. If it failed the first time, it will probably fail the subsequent times too. That said then, we need a new strategy. When you concentrate on the quality instead of the quantity you will be choosing good wholesome foods instead of high fat snack type foods.

We will be examining "wholefoods" in more detail later in the course. But as a taster (pardon the pun) the types of food we are talking about here is potatoes, pasta, beans, whole grains etc.

When you're buying food, consideration ought to be made to the quality of the food. Cheapest is not always the best, as we well know. It is often quoted "You get what you pay for". This is normally used for all goods in general but is especially relevant when it comes to the stuff we put into our faces. When it comes to meat products, lean fillet is better than a cheap fatty cut but as we all know and appreciate, this is not always the viable option given financial restraint. That said though, it is usually false economy to always go for the cheapest cut of meat as there could be a lot of waste with the gristle and unwanted fat.

COME ON!

- It's cardio day again. Time to get out of breath and re-energise the brain.
- Don't forget to mix it up a bit.

Break your records!

#44. DRIVING YOU NUTS

The car is a place where a lot of people struggle to keep temptation out of reach. There are very few (if any) garages that do not sell an abundance of sweets and crisps etc. It is therefore a potential minefield for those who are vulnerable. Always have plenty of fruit, nuts, seeds etc in the car so you don't get tempted by the crisps and chocolate. For your own and everyone's safety you should not be eating while you drive anyway, as the police will gladly tell you, which is a great reason not to.

Also have water in the car. Make it a habit to drink some water before you set off and when you arrive at your destination. The car is probably most people's downfall when it comes to unhealthy eating. Boredom can take the pennies out of your pocket and into the cashier's hand quicker than lightning. Be prepared. Before you enter the garage shop, take a swig of your nice fresh water to quash some of the imaginary hunger.

Today's new resistance exercise is the "Bicep Curl". This exercise will build up the muscle on the front of your upper arm.

FBI Bicep Curl

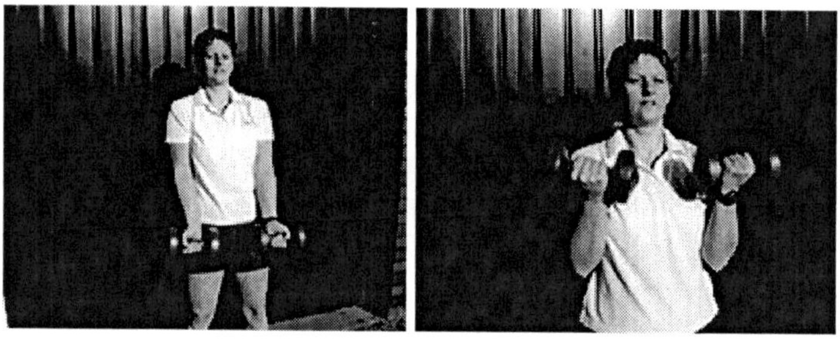

Holding your weights at your side, ensure that your upper arm remains still throughout the movement. Bend the elbows and bring the weights up to your shoulders. Return the weights under control back down to your sides. Breathe out on the way up.

COME ON!

- Add the “Bicep Curl” to your Training Program 2 x 10.
- Carry out the full resistance program.

Feel the strength getting better each time.

#45. HULK OR HULKESS?

Congratulations, you have reached the halfway stage of the course and you're still working at it. Today I'm going to talk about muscle mass and how to build it. But first, I'll dispel a myth.

Females don't go big and bulky with weight training. It is the male hormone testosterone, which is responsible for this. Ladies will just increase the leanness of the muscle, which gives the muscle good definition.

Fear of bulking up is one reason why some ladies shy away from weight training. Remember that lean muscle burns the calories, so the more muscles that you can get lean and strong the more calories you will burn, even at rest.

To build muscle mass, we need to train the muscle hard and out of its comfort zone. The way we do this is to work the muscle to failure. The amount of repetitions we do is between 8 and 12. If you can do more than 12 reps then the weight you are lifting is too light.

If you want to maximise muscle growth you'll have to increase the weight. Ladies, don't get scared, remember you will not get like a hulkess as it's the testosterone that does this. You will get more defined muscles though and get stronger by the session.

Subsequently, if you cannot do 8 before failure, then the weight is too heavy and you need to reduce the weight. We want these muscles to get really fatigued so they build up (Hypertrophy) in recovery and get stronger. You may need to purchase a new set of dumbbells if you are finding the exercises too easy. Investment in your strength is worthwhile because the stronger you are now, the stronger you'll be when you get older. However, if you do not want to increase the size of your muscles you can stick with the same weights. Remember you own the Training Program.

COME ON!

- Change the following exercises to 2 x 8 - 12
- Lateral Raise, Upright Row, Shoulder Press
- Change the Tricep Dips to 2 x Fatigue
- Change the following exercises to 2 x 20
    - Squats
    - Lunges
    - Vee Sits
- We have not changed the Bicep curl as it is a relatively new exercise.

No exercise today, but look forward to your next (hard) resistance session.

#46. DON'T PUNISH YOURSELF

If you think I'm going soft on you, think again. This one is for the mind. If you've faltered on your healthy lifestyle whether it is eating too much rubbish or not training enough, then correct it now.

Don't beat yourself up over what has passed. It's gone forever and you can't change that. Just get on with the job in hand. Things aren't generally irreversible and all that would have happened is you will have slipped back a pace.

The main thing is that you come back on track as soon as you can. Use this as a training session in itself. Identify what it was that made you slip and see if you can put a strategy in place to stop it happening again.

Too many people dwell too long on what has passed and I've heard so many people say "well I've ruined it now, I may as well forget it!" Stop yourself if you ever hear yourself say this. Nothing is lost. If you didn't relapse some of the time, then you probably wouldn't be doing this course in the first place. Forward thinking and forward action. The fact that you are still here after 46 days is enough proof that you really want this.

If on the other hand you have managed to keep to all your schedules, well done you. Feel good about yourself for all your persistence and hard work.

COME ON!

- Time to up the cardio again.
- Make your cardio session now last 30 minutes.
- This would make the whole session last for 45 minutes broken down as follows.
    - Warm-up 10 mins
    - Main Session 30 mins
    - Cool-down & Stretch 5 mins

Increase the rest periods in your skipping and straddles to one minute. This is so that you can really "go for it". Remember, you would now be up to 15 intervals. Or, you could do half and half. The choice is yours.

Remember to always record your results. They should be looking pretty impressive by now.

#47. THE PULL-UP

Today's exercise is a very difficult one.

This doesn't mean it should be avoided though, on the contrary we are going for it big style.

The first problem involved with the pull-up is where to do it. You do need a firm and secure overhead bar or beam on which to do this. If you're a member of a gym, you might have a purpose built bar with which to do it but for the rest of us, a touch of improvisation is required.

I use the rafters in my garage if I'm at home. I acquired an old "pull-down" bar from an old multigym and put it over the rafters. I also have in the past just used the bare rafters.

Those with soft hands, remember that a pair of gloves might be wise here. If I'm out and about running, I usually find something that I can hang off. Just make sure that it is legal and safe to use whatever you find.

Talking of this, as I run through an area, I'm always on the lookout for bits of natural equipment that I can use for training. From a bench to a cut log. Anything is fair game for me.

FBI Pull-Up

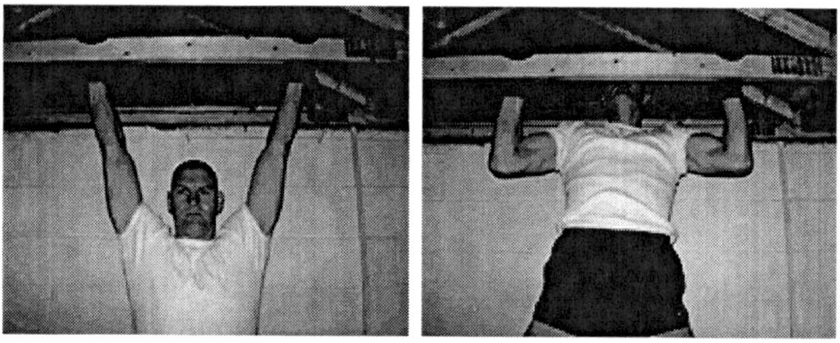

- Use a wide overhand grip and let your body hang down naturally.
- Pull up your body until your chin reaches the bar.

- Lower back down until your arms are fully extended as in the starting position.

I told you it was difficult. If you are training in pairs one can assist the other in the upward movement. The "puller" crosses their feet behind their body and the "helper" assists by putting their hands under the "pullers" legs and lifting.

Don't be too put off if you still find it incredibly difficult. You can only get better. This exercise works your Latissimus Dorsi (the Lats), which are the muscles at the sides of your back under your arms. When these muscles are developed it gives the body that "Vee" look.

COME ON!

- Add the "Pull-up" to your training program - 2 x to fatigue.
- Carry out the rest of your session as per your program.
- This should be quite a hard session but I know you're ready for it.

#48. RECIPE FOR SUCCESS

We all like to experiment from time to time and with food it should be no different.

When trying out new recipes, try cutting half the butter, salt, sugar or cream etc from the ingredients. Some of the outcomes will not be affected and who knows, you may prefer the taste and it will be healthier.

You can always add more as you go on. This is the beauty of cooking or baking for yourself. You are in control of the ingredients, which will help you to keep your "Food Diary" pretty accurate. As well as cutting down on some products, you can also add your favourites in there too to make it more tasty.

Be prepared for the odd disaster, I've served up a pretty mean fruit smoothie in my time that just didn't go. But then I've created many a nice fruit bread which you just couldn't buy. Experimenting is all about successes and the odd failure, go on, give it a go.

COME ON!

- Pick a new or favourite recipe from a book or magazine.
- Alter the ingredients to make it healthier.
- Share your secret.

Happy cooking.

#49. "ON YER BIKE!"

As we arrive at another day for your cardio-vascular training, I'm going to mention cycling.

Whether you cycle out doors or on a static bike at the gym or your home is regardless. They will all do you a lot of good. Getting outdoors in the fresh air (if you live in a smog filled city, you might have to go further afield) is the best, fighting against the elements.

Certain things can put you off with outdoor cycling I do appreciate that. Bad weather for a start (If you're in the UK that is), busy traffic is another. This is where the static bikes have an advantage, but if you get on a good cycle path, a planned route maybe, then it just doesn't compare. If you like a bit of company when you cycle, again it's difficult if you're cycling round the streets. But all that said, the principle is the same.

If you want to improve your heart and lungs along with your leg strength, then you have to be prepared to put some hard graft in. Just as in jogging where you are trying to beat your best each time, you need to be working outside your comfort zone for maximum benefit.

Once you've got used to being in the saddle find some good hills on your route to increase your intensity. Off road cycling is more difficult still. So as you can see there is a good variety for those who may be beginners on a bike or those who have cycled a fair bit in the past.

COME ON!

- Add cycling to your training program.
- Even if you prefer to do the running, skipping or straddle jumps, it's always good to have a bit of variety.

Get on your bike!

#50. DINNER LIKE A PAUPER

I spoke before on Breakfast like a King, lunch like a Prince. The remaining one is "Dinner like a Pauper". This is because we are generally in "wind down" mode (or should be) after dinner. Therefore we do not need as many calories to sustain us through this time of the day.

Our culture though has changed and we tend to save our big meal of the day for dinnertime to coincide with the family coming together again after a day's work. It is a healthy practice to all sit down as a family for dinner, but it can be healthier if we cut down on the intake at this time.

A lot of people save themselves for this meal and go hungry all day, which as we've proved already in the course is not good practice. Not only does it mean that you save your entire calorie intake for the time of day when your body doesn't really want or need them but by going hungry all day you leave yourself vulnerable for the high fat/sugar snacks to tide you over. On top of that, being hungry is not pleasant and it is totally unnecessary.

The next exercise for your resistance program is the "Calf Raise". This exercise is for the back of the lower leg. The only thing you need for this is a step.

FBI Calf Raise

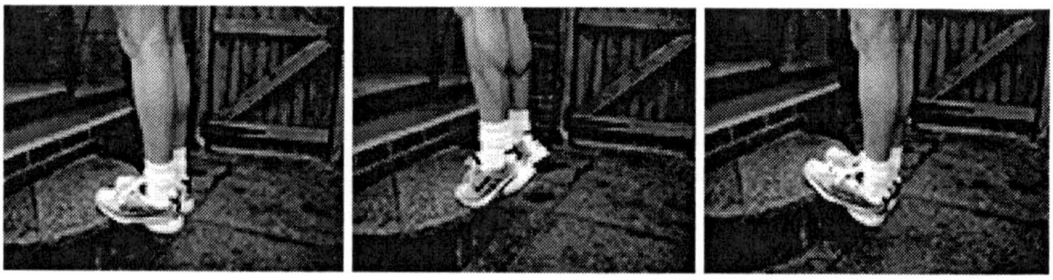

1. Stand with your toes on the step, you may want to hold on to something to get your balance at first.
2. Lift up onto your "tip-toes" and hold it for a couple of seconds
3. Then lower until your heel is well below the step

4. You should also feel the calf muscle stretch as you reach the bottom of the movement.

When you get to the stage when it gets a bit easy, you can lift one leg and carry out the exercise on one leg at a time.

COME ON!

- It's your resistance session today.
- Add the Calf Raises to your workout. 2 x 20 should suffice for the first go.
- Do you have enough time scheduled for a whole session?
- It takes me about an hour to do it all with a minute in between each set.

We'll look at splitting the session into two in the next resistance session to allow you to either do more on a specific muscle or to save you a bit of time. Remember, the choice will be yours.

#51. MORAL FIBRE

Are you getting enough fibre in your diet? Do you know the job of fibre in your body? Well let's start with what it is. Fibre (or non starch polysaccharides) is the indigestible plant material such as cellulose, lignin and pectin, which is found in fruits, vegetables, grains and beans. It doesn't contain any nutrients, although it is vital to a healthy body since it usually comes wrapped around valuable foods, as well as being important in its own right.

It provides bulk to your food, helps the food pass easily along the gut and absorbs water. It is not lost in the cooking process. There are two basic types of fibre:

Insoluble - A woody, structural part of the plant for example fruit, vegetable skins, wheat, rye and corn. It:

1. Does not dissolve in water.
2. Passes through the gut unchanged.
3. Aids peristalsis, which speeds the passage of food.
4. Reduces the risk of some colon cancers.
5. Carries excess fat with it.

Soluble - Found in beans, barley, oats, broccoli, prunes, apples and citrus fruits. It:

1. Dissolves in water
2. Has a consistency of a gel
3. Lowers blood cholesterol.
4. Helps to regulate blood sugar

So as you can see, it's very important that we should be getting our correct quota of the stuff. It also helps to understand what happens to the fibre in our body.

In the mouth - Fibre is very bulky and satisfying to eat. It takes a lot longer to chew, which releases more saliva that is good for your dental health.

In the stomach - High fibre food is in the stomach for about 2 hours. Low fibre food is there for less time. Therefore a high fibre meal seems more satisfying and prevents us from feeling hungry after eating.

In the small intestine - High fibre food has a thick sticky consistency, and can help to slow down the absorption of sugar into the blood. This reduces the demands on the pancreas to release insulin. Fruit and vegetables may help prevent cholesterol and fat from being absorbed in the small intestine, which, in turn, can help to prevent heart disease and assist weight loss.

In the large intestine - Fibre gathers with waste food products and water. Together, they form a bulky, moist stool, which can pass smoothly, easily and relatively quickly from the body.

In the rectum and anus - With a high fibre diet the stools will pass out of the body relatively quickly and without any discomfort.

It is imperative though to make sure if you have a high fibre diet, you also ensure that your water intake is also at least 2 litres daily. If not, then the fibre can actually bung you up reversing many of the good qualities that it's being consumed for.

As this is a big subject, I will explain the benefits of a high fibre diet tomorrow.

COME ON!

- Rest day from exercise today.
- Time to catch up on the bits and pieces that you may have let slip (if any of course).
- Check the fibre content in your daily diet by having a look at the food labels - it should be approx 18g.

Happy hunting!

#52. MORE MORAL FIBRE

Yesterday I told you about the importance of fibre within the diet. Today we'll look at the benefits of a high fibre diet, when taken with adequate water.

Reduced Constipation - As referred to yesterday, the bulk of the fibre, plus the water and bacteria added to the waste, produce a stool consistency, which is much easier to remove from the body without straining. Since the straining associated with constipation might be linked to haemorrhoids, hernias and varicose veins, a high fibre diet can also prevent these problems. It can help to prevent (and to relieve) irritable bowel syndrome (alternating diarrhoea and constipation).

Reduced Heart Disease - Soluble fibre helps to reduce the blood cholesterol level when a high fibre intake is taken by people with high cholesterol.

Regulates Blood Sugar Levels - Soluble fibre regulates blood sugar levels by slowing down sugar absorption in the intestines. This is of particular benefit to diabetics.

Reduced Risk of Bowel Cancer - Some of the fibre in our diet is broken down by bacteria, to produce special substances, which may prevent the lining of the colon being affected by carcinogens.

Reduced Incidence of Gallstones - Some studies suggest that gallstones are more common in diabetics, overweight people and people with low fibre diets. Gallstones are often accumulations of the cholesterol that is in the bile. Eating more soluble fibre can reduce the amount of cholesterol in the bile.

Reduced Weight - Eating more fibre is supposed to make weight loss easier. This is because it:

- Takes longer to eat.
- Stays longer in the stomach so is more filling.
- Slows down the absorption of sugars.
- Carries more fat through the body so we excrete more calories.

Whether the fuller feeling is psychological or real (because of the extra time it takes to eat high fibre foods) fibre certainly seems to make weight loss an easier process. A high fibre diet is frequently low in fat and sugar too.

How much do you need?

Yesterday I mentioned that you need about 18 grams of fibre. To encourage you to gradually increase your intake of fibre to 18g a day (if it isn't already), it would be good to know what 18g looks like in respect of typical foods. These are approximate measures and to be taken with at least 2 litres of water.

2 Shredded Wheat = 3.0 g

1 Banana = 1.8 g

1 Apple = 1.2 g

1 Portion of Broccoli = 2.4 g

4 Slices of Wholemeal Bread = 7.2 g

1 Jacket Potato = 2.4 g

Total = **18 g**

Or another would be

2 Weetabix = 2.7 g

1 small tin of Baked Beans = 4.8 g

2 Slices Wholemeal Bread = 3.6 g

28g of Dried Apricots = 4.5 g

1 Jacket Potato = 2.4 g

Total = **18 g**

COME ON!

- How did your daily intake match up to examples?
- If it's way out, time to put in the changes.
- Cardio session today.
- Pick one of the activities that you haven't done for a while.
- See if you've improved. You should have.

Oh, and always remember to record your results!

#53. LET'S TWIST AGAIN

Toady we are going to twist the torso into shape.

The muscles that we are going to exercise are the "Obliques". These are your side abdominals responsible for bending the body to the side. We are also going to split the resistance program into 2 different sessions.

As you progress and start to increase the number of sets you perform for each exercise, the sheer volume of work could become unmanageable and too time consuming. Split routines, whereby different muscles are exercised on different days, allow a greater volume of work to be performed on these muscle groups while also allowing adequate recovery times.

Resistance session 1 will be, Chest/Back/Shoulders.

Resistance session 2 will be Arms/Legs/Abdominals

This is only a rough guide, as the arms for instance will also work when you're working your chest and shoulders.

So, now to the new exercise. The "Torso Twist":

FBI Torso Twist

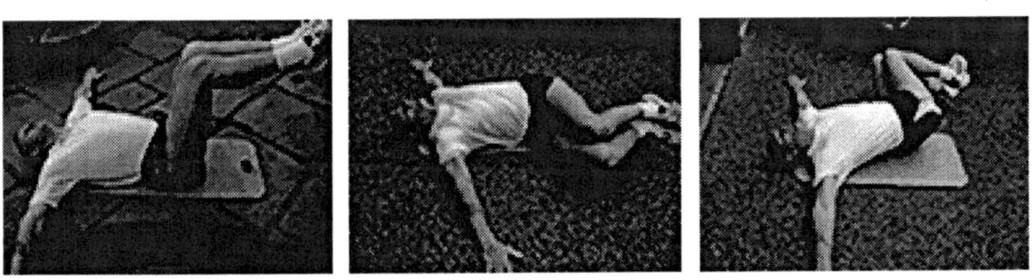

1. Lie down on your mat and lift your legs until your hips and knees are at right angles.
2. Stretch out your arms to the side and keep your shoulders on the floor.

3. Keeping your upper body stationary on the mat, rotate your hips so your knees move towards the floor, first one side and then the other.
4. Don't worry if you don't reach the floor at first, you will get better the more you do the exercise.

COME ON!

- Split your resistance into the following two sessions.
    1. Session 1: Press-ups 3 x fatigue, Lateral Raise 3 x 8-12, Upright Row 3 x 8-12, Shoulder Press 3 x 8-12, Pull-ups 3 x fatigue, Dorsal Raises 3 x 10
    2. Session 2: Squats 3 x 20, Lunges 3 x 20, Calf Raises 3 x 20, Tricep Dips 3 x fatigue, Bicep Curls 3 x 8-12, Crunches 3 x 10, Vee Sits 3 x 20. Torso Twists 3 x 20 (10 each side)
- You may have noticed that I have increased your sets to 3. This is all part of the progressing procedure.
- Add your Torso Twist and start with session 2 today.

Go for it, work hard!

#54. CEREALS AND WHOLEGRAINS

Today we are going to look at "Cereals" and "Wholegrains". So, what are they? Think of cereals and we usually think of breakfast, but really they are the edible seeds or grains of the grass family. These are:

- Oats
- Barley
- Wheat
- Rye
- Maize (Corn)
- Brown Rice
- Millet

The term "wholegrain" means that all 3 parts of the grain are present in the food. These are:

The Bran - This is the "fibre rich" outer layer, which is also called the husk. This layer is full of fibre, B vitamins, 50 to 80% of the grain's minerals and other health promoting plant substances called "phytochemicals".

The Endosperm - The "starchy" middle. This portion is full of complex carbohydrates, protein and smaller amounts of B vitamins.

The Germ - "nutrient packed", the germ is full of B vitamins, vitamin E, trace minerals, and healthy unsaturated fats, phytochemicals and antioxidants.

Nothing has been taken out in the food processing stage so all the goodness is still there.

When the germ and bran portions are removed during milling, the nutrient content is reduced by 25 to 95%. Most refined grain foods are enriched with some of the nutrients lost in milling. This will generally be seen on the label as "Fortified with". It is not unlike being "mugged" for your wallet and given enough money back for your bus fare.

Beware of fancy names that don't mean wholegrain. Some of the more popular ones are:

- 100% wheat - means only that the only grain is wheat. It may not contain whole wheat.
- Multigrain - A word that means the product contains more than one kind of grain. The food may not however contain whole grains.
- Granary - Another term that does not signify the use of whole grains.

I've said it before but it's always worth repeating. Food eaten in its natural state is far better than when it has been processed. It is as nature intended.

COME ON!

- It's back to your cupboards again today.
- Check out your cereals.
- See how many wholegrains as opposed to refined products you have in there.

Be aware the next time you do your shopping.

#55. GET FRUITY

Fruit like our own body consists of over 70% water. It is packed with fibre, natural sugars, vitamins and minerals. It is the most natural of all foods growing unaided in some parts of the world for centuries.

Different coloured fruits contain different properties, therefore as was mentioned in lesson 40 we should eat a rainbow. We should be eating at least 5 portions of fruit a day. It is difficult to overeat when it comes to fruit.

Fruit is the ultimate in "fast foods". If you've ever heard someone say that they haven't got time to eat healthy hit them with this challenge. To grab a so called "fast meal" while you grab some fruit and see who is eating first. Somehow I think you will have finished while they are still being served.

Fruits are easy to eat and are mostly an excellent convenience food. I say mostly as my favourite fruit is ripe succulent mango, which is anything but convenient unless you are standing naked in a bath.

COME ON!

- Are you eating a rainbow? Time to get on board again if you've let it slip.
- It's a cardio day today, let's get out of breath and make some positive progress.

Always remember to warm-up and cool-down properly.

#56. THINK POSITIVELY

Have you ever had those nagging doubts that you'll never get there or you won't succeed? Why I wonder...

This is an area that could cover more than a dozen days so I'm only going to say, "think positively about all you do". This is a bit like how the placebo effect works, you think it's doing you good so you feel better. It's the "feeling better", which will promote the healing qualities of your own body. If you think things will happen they generally will, so start to think positively and see the changes come to fruition.

Beliefs are not reality. A belief is an emotion, a feeling of certainty about something. This belief can be empowering or dis-empowering. A belief is built up through reinforcement, and any pattern of emotion or behaviour that is continually reinforced will become an automatic and conditioned response.

So if you believe you are not able to do a task, you will probably be right. Change the way you think and see the difference it will make. Walk like you are already fit and healthy. Talk as if you are fit and healthy and most of all believe that you are fit and healthy. Live the dream and the dream will become reality.

In honour of someone always thinking positive, today's exercise is called the "Superman". Christopher Reeve never gave up thinking positive through all his adversity. He was always looking at new ways to improve his life.

The "Superman" works the lower back muscles and generally improves your inner core muscles and balance.

FBI Superman

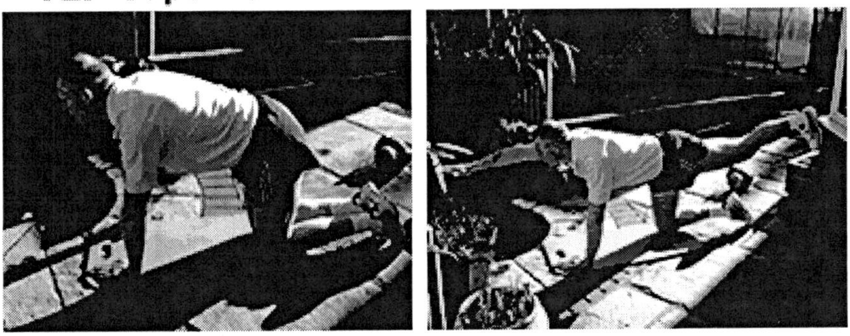

1. Kneel on all fours. Keep a neutral spine and tense your abdominal muscles throughout the exercise.
2. Outstretch your left arm and right leg together.
3. Hold them straight and still for 20 seconds.
4. Change sides and exercise the right arm and left leg together.

As a progression to this exercise, close your eyes, which takes out one of your senses that assist you in balancing.

COME ON!

- Add the "Superman" (3 x each side) to your resistance training program.
- Carry out session 1 of the resistance program.

Feel the difference!

#57. GOOD FAT BAD FAT

Fats represent the most concentrated forms of energy in our diet. They yield nine calories of energy per gram, when oxidised compared with only four calories per gram from proteins and carbohydrates.

Fats generally get bad press for one reason or another but they are essential for the normal functioning of the body. The main functions of fats in the body are:

- To protect body organs
- Provide insulation
- Protect the brain
- Coat the nerves in a myelin sheath
- Important carriers of vitamins A, D, E and K into the body
- To give the body shape (sometimes too much)
- Reserve energy source

Fats and oils are both fats. The difference can be generally described as follows.

Fat - Saturated Fat

Usually solid at room temperature. Saturated fats mainly come from an animal source. This is usually regarded as the "bad fat" and should be limited to only about 6% of your diet.

Too much saturated fat is linked with a higher risk of coronary heart disease as it has been proved to raise blood cholesterol levels. The food labels will point out how much saturated fat that there is in the particular food. This is the one to keep an eye on.

Oil - Unsaturated Fat

Usually liquid at room temperature. Unsaturated fats come mainly from a vegetable or oily fish source. These fats are generally known as the "good fats" and should make up about 14% of the diet.

Unsaturated fats are usually known as the healthy fats, the ones that we should be taking in, but careful here, as some unsaturated fats are a lot healthier than others.

Monounsaturated fatty acids that are found in Olive oil, Rapeseed oil and Peanut oil are healthy fats. Use sparingly though as the calorie count is high with fats. Polyunsaturated fatty acids found in Sunflower oil or seeds, Safflower oil and Corn oil are also a good healthy fat.

Unsaturated fatty acids can also be “cis” or “trans”. A “cis” fatty acid is a natural fatty acid, which you would find in a good cold pressed olive oil. In the unheated state this oil is very beneficial to your health. A “trans” fatty acid though is an unnatural fatty acid as found in hydrogenated margarines. This fat is not beneficial to health. A “cis” fatty acid can be converted to a “trans” fatty acid through the process of hydrogenation or heating.

So, as you can see, fat is not so straight forward as it seems. Food labels will tell you what kind of fat that the food includes. The ingredients will also let you know if the unhealthy fats are present. Remember though, we do need a certain amount of fat within the diet. Just ensure that the ones you get are the healthy ones.

In the next session we’ll look at some tips to cut down on your fat content (if you need to of course).

COME ON!

- Back to your food cupboard and fridge.
- Check out your labels and see what kind of fats you are taking in.
- Are you surprised at what you see? I hope not.

More fat busting tomorrow!

#58. FAT CUTTING TIPS

Today is your Cardio-Vascular day and I hope that you are truly feeling the benefits of all the exercise by now. The feeling will just get better and better believe me.

Also today we are looking at simple tips to reducing the fat content in your diet if it is too high. This is where your food diary becomes invaluable. Knowing what goes in enables us to adjust the intake accordingly. Without this we would only be guessing. If you are already spot on with your fat content then I applaud you but I feel some of you may need these tips to assist you on your journey.

- Bin the deep fat fryer. Grilling, boiling, poaching and steaming are healthier ways of cooking your food.
- If you are frying, try using a non-stick pan and as little oil as possible and get rid of the lard.
- Choose lean cuts of meat and trim off all visible fat.
- Eat less meat and replace with fresh vegetables.
- Reduce pies and pastry products.
- Eat fewer chips and french fries. If you cook them, cut them thick and straight or use oven chips.
- Eat fish more often. Grill, steam or bake it rather than fry it in batter.
- Make salad dressings with natural yoghurt, herbs, spices, tomato juice, vinegar or lemon juice rather than using mayonnaise or salad cream.
- Chicken and Turkey are low in fat if cooked without the skin on.
- Use butter but spread it very thinly.
- Reduce meat products like beefburgers, sausages etc. If you do use them think quality over quantity. Read the labels carefully and choose foods that are lower in fat.
- Be careful with "low fat" products as some of them are packed with more sugar to compensate for the lack of fat to improve the taste.

Most of the tips are simple and obvious, but then again most good things in life are simple.

Rowing is a great cardio exercise but is often limited to gym users. We are going to add it to our list of cardio exercises as I know some of you are using the gym or have home equipment. If you haven't got access to a rowing machine, you can still carry on with your other cardio exercises. The principle is still the same though as we are striving to work out of our comfort zone and improve on our performance.

When we row we need to follow a few basic guidelines. Breathe out when you are on the pulling stroke. Do not hyper-extend the knees (don't lock them out). Keep your arms straight until your hands are level with your knees, then, pull your hands into your midriff.

COME ON!

- Add Rowing into your cardio session - 10 minutes duration.
- Integrate rowing into your routine if possible.
- Progress and record your results in whatever cardio activity you decide to do today.
- You should now be looking to prolong your cardio session to 35 minutes.
- This means that you should now be on a 50 minute cardio workout including your warm up and stretching routine.
- For variation and an added intensity, combine skipping with straddles, and add hand weights when you do your straddles.

Go for it!

#59. STEP LIGHTLY

Today's new exercise involves the use of a box. It is called the "Step Over".

It is better if the box is adjustable in height but don't worry if it's not as long as what you are using is steady on the floor. This is a good cross training type exercise as it also dips into your cardio vascular system making it an ideal exercise for "circuit training".

FBI Step Over

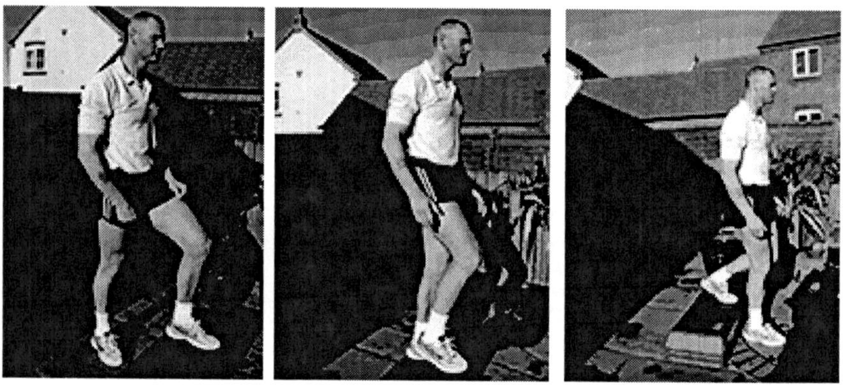

1. The starting position is standing behind your box with your left foot placed flat on the middle of the box.
2. Next, shift your weight onto your left leg and step fully over the box, placing your right foot squarely on the floor in front of the box.
3. You now push back down with your left leg and lift your right leg back over to the rear of the box, just like in the starting position. This completes one rep keeping the left leg on the box for the rest of the required reps.
4. Now it's time to swap the legs over, putting your right foot in the middle of the box. Repeat the format with your opposite leg.

For progression you can raise the height of your box (or get a bigger object to step onto). You will definitely feel a burn with these when you get going.

COME ON!

- Add the "Step Overs" to your resistance session 2. Two sets of 10 reps on each leg at first. Only use body weight for now until you get used to it.
- Carry out the rest of your resistance session number 2.

Feel those muscles building with each session.

#60. SUPPLEMENTARY EVIDENCE

Today's topic is the sometimes controversial subject of supplements.

Some dieticians would tell you that you could get all the nutrients you need from a well balanced diet. On the other hand some of them would tell you that intense over farming has lowered the level of nutrients that are expected in food, and due to lifestyle in general, most people would benefit from a basic multi-vitamin or mineral supplement.

So, which opinion do you agree with?

Here are some views for and against supplementation.

For

- If a deficiency of a vitamin/mineral is established by someone suitably qualified.
- Classes of people who need to improve nutritional status e.g. vegetarians who omit a whole food group.
- Some people may need supplements to reduce disease risk e.g. post menopausal women may wish to supplement their calcium intake to deter osteoporosis.
- Special circumstances could create a need for dietary supplements. An example is women who lose a lot of blood during menstruation each month may feel they need an iron supplement.
- Appropriate supplementation may be necessary to overcome surgery or disease to improve the body's immune system.

Against

- Taking individual supplements can cause other imbalances.
- Toxicity - the extent and severity of supplement toxicity remain unclear.
- There are no guarantees that supplements will be effective.
- They can be expensive - some people may spend a lot of money on supplements thinking they are superior to food,

and not leave enough money for the buying of real food. This may lead to a false sense of security regarding nutrition and problems involving disordered eating patterns.
- Supplements can't supply energy.

So now you're wondering what side of the fence I'm on. Sorry guys I'm on the fence on this one as there are benefits to taking supplements so long as you are sure that you cannot get the particular vitamin or mineral from food alone. Supplements are what they say they are, they supplement a diet, they don't replace it.

I will leave you with a fact. The body can't store extra vitamins, so if you have had enough through food then the extra is just discharged by the body through the urine.

COME ON!

- A rest day from exercise.
- List all the supplements that you take at present.
- Scrutinise the list along with your food diary and see, which ones are not really necessary.

The bottom line is, ALWAYS know what you're taking and WHY.

#61. AVOID THE FADS

There are lots of "fad" diets out there promising you the body that you desire for seemingly little work from you. Like most things in life you get out what you put in. Put little effort in and you will get little results out.

Some of the fads are based on a normal eating plan with a twist. Some encourage the cutting out of whole food groups, which deprive the body of vital nutrients. The shelves are full of different types of fads from Blood Group, F Plan, GI diet, Atkins, Cabbage soup etc etc. We could go on forever and I bet some of you have had a go at them all. So if you have and you're here, why is that, did they fail? They usually do.

Celebrities often hold up one of these as the reason they are looking slim. Ask the question, does that celebrity always look good? Ever seen the pictures of them without make-up? Their skin doesn't look too good to me. A healthy glow is borne out of natural food and a good healthy lifestyle. Putting your name to a product is big bucks so don't be taken in by celebrity endorsements.

Some clubs offer you the chance to go along and get weighed for a price every week. This is a brilliant plan, wish I had thought of that one. I do know private clubs where a half a dozen friends and family all get together once a week, put in five pounds and the one who has lost the most collects the pot. At least that way the money goes to someone you like.

This 90 day course as you will have gathered by now is not a fad. It is a sustainable lifestyle that you are in control of tweaking it when and where you need to. With the knowledge you are gaining you control your destiny. Stick with it and put the effort in. You will be pleased with the eventual outcome.

COME ON!

- Cardio day again.
- How is your progress going? Are you trying out different cardio sessions?
- Whichever one you do, always remember to record the results and compare them to when you first did that particular session.

See you tomorrow.

#62. LEARN TO FLY

Today we're going to learn to fly. Well okay not quite fly but "Flye". These are resistance exercises for the pectorals (chest muscles). You need some sort of a bench for this exercise along with your weights. Talking of weights, are you increasing your weights when you find that you can do 12 reps? If not you could be losing out on valuable muscle building opportunities. Always remember, lean muscle burns more calories, even when they are at rest.

So, to the exercise:

FBI Flye

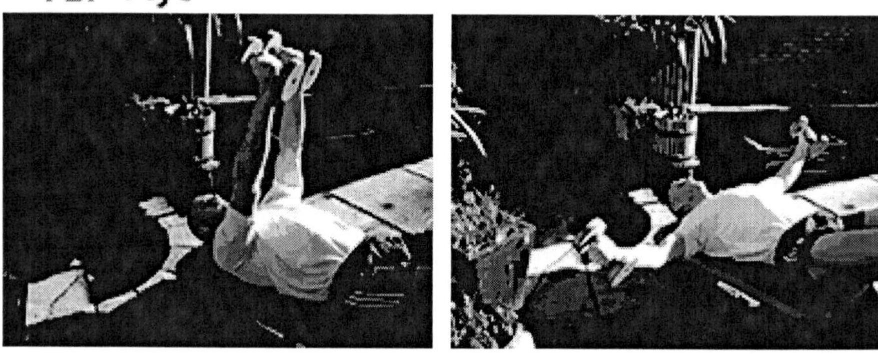

1. Lie down on the bench with your weights down on your chest. Keep your feet flat on the floor.
2. Lift up the weights until your arms are fully extended without locking the elbows.
3. Keeping your back flat on the bench and maintaining the angle at your elbows, bring your arms down in an arc until your elbows are level with the middle line of your body.
4. Breathing out as you bring the weights back up through the same arc to the top again (as in the first photo).
5. That completes one rep.

If you feel your arms moving inwards changing the angle at your elbows, the weight is too heavy for you. Strict form throughout the exercise will ensure you get the maximum benefit.

This exercise, for variation, can be done at an incline or a decline. This alters the emphasis slightly on the working muscles bringing an extended range of muscle fibres into play. For example you will recruit the upper fibres of the pectorals in an incline and the lower fibres in a decline position. Try it out to see the difference.

COME ON!

- Add the “Flyes” to your resistance session number 1 with a rep range of 3 x 10 with light weights for starters.
- Carry out session 1 in its entirety.

Work hard!

#63. COMPLEX CARBS

Carbohydrates have been getting quite a bit of bashing lately, much of it uncalled for I might add. It is not just "too many carbs" that make you overweight, it is over eating in general and a lack of adequate exercise. "Calories in" versus "calories out" regardless of where they come from.

So let's look at what a carbohydrate is and where the best sources are in our food chain.

Carbohydrate is the name given to a group of foods from "simple sugars" to the more complex carbohydrates such as "starches" and "fibres". It is the body's preferred source of fuel. Simple sugars are known as Monosaccharides (one sugar). If two saccharides are joined together they form Disaccharides and many saccharides joined together are called Polysaccharides. During digestion, enzymes break down the disaccharides and polysaccharides into the simple monosaccharide of Glucose, which can then be absorbed into the bloodstream.

A complex carbohydrate needs a lot of digestive enzymatic action in order to break it down to a usable source of fuel (glucose) for the body. Because it takes longer to break down a complex carb, it releases the energy slowly therefore avoiding a quick rise in your blood sugar level also called a "sugar spike".

Good sources of carbohydrates are whole grains (see day #54), which contain vitamins, minerals protein and some oils, which are important for good nutrition. Others include potatoes, bananas, beans, peas, lentils and leguminous vegetables.

A total lack of carbohydrate or very low intake may produce a condition called Ketosis. Ketosis is accompanied by muscular weakness, fatigue, nausea, headache, dizziness, confusion, irritability, anxiety and a marked decline in performance. Not a desirable state to be in but some do it in an effort to lose weight. The body in this state will burn fat and muscle protein for energy.

As we know now, get rid of the muscle and we get rid of our calorie burning potential.

COME ON!

- Have a look at your food diary and see where you are getting all your carbohydrate from.
- You are now seeing the importance of the food diary as we re-visit it regularly.

I will delve into the "simple sugars" very shortly. By then though, you should be getting into the complex carb way of life

#64. USE A HEART RATE MONITOR

Have you ever thought about using a Heart Rate Monitor (HRM)? Well it can be a very useful ally during your training sessions. When I used one it helped me to improve my running times substantially without ever getting to the stage of total exhaustion.

First of all you need to find out what your Maximum Heart Rate (MHR) is. There is an easy calculation to find an approximate reading. It is:

```
220 Minus Your Age
```

Simple as that. So if a person aged 45 was training, their MHR would be...

```
220 - 45 = 175 beats per minute
```

This then is their guide to how hard they can work their heart. This is only a guide though and you may be able to work quite a few beats above your reading quite comfortably.

Taking your reading, you now work out how hard you want to work. I prefer to work hard when I am running or carrying out cardio work and therefore use a range between 80% and 95% of my MHR. How I use my HRM is when I'm warmed up I run until my HRM reads 95% (for me it is 166), then I slow down until my heart rate falls to 85% (149), then up the pace again. That is the way I use my monitor. If you train to run fast you will be a good fast runner, train slow and you will become a good slow runner. Play around with your figures until you find a level where you are working hard without hitting total exhaustion.

COME ON!

- It's a cardio day today.
- Use a different cardio exercise today to keep the brain stimulated.
- Record your results.

Look back at when you first started and see the difference. Inspiring or what?

#65. CHECK YOUR PULSE

How do you know how hard you are working? If you use a HRM as talked about yesterday it's easy, you just look at the watch. Another method is to check your own pulse. It's very quick and easy to do especially when you're doing interval training.

To check your pulse

- Place your index and middle finger over the underside of your opposite wrist, below the base of the thumb. If it is hard to feel the pulse in your wrist, place your index and middle finger just to the side of your Adam's apple, in the soft hollow area at the side of your neck.
- With the flat part of your fingers rather than the tips, press firmly, but not so hard that you can't feel the pulse. If you are taking someone else's pulse, do not use your thumb or you will feel your own pulse along with the other person's.
- Count the number of beats for 30 seconds, then, multiply that number by 2 to get the beats per minute. Or count the number of beats for 15 seconds, then, multiply by 4 to get the beats per minute. If you are taking your pulse during exercise, you may count the beats for only 10 seconds and multiply by 6. The most accurate way is to count the beats for the whole minute.

Normal resting heart rate

Many factors affect normal heart rate, including your age, activity level, and the time of day. The chart below shows the normal range of a resting heart rate (pulse rate after resting 10 minutes) in beats per minute, according to age. In general, the lower your resting heart rate, the more efficient your heart is and the healthier you are. The best time to take this is before you get out of bed in the morning.

Age/Fitness Level	Resting Heart Rate Beats per minute (bpm)
Babies to age 1:	100-160
Children ages 1 to 10:	60-140
Children/Adults age 10+:	60-100
Well-conditioned athletes:	40-60

Your pulse usually has a steady or regular rhythm. An occasional pause or extra beat is normal. Talk to your health professional if you notice frequent skipped or extra beats and it's causing you some concern. Normally, your heart rate increases slightly when you inhale deeply and drops slightly as you exhale. You can check this normal change in your pulse rate by changing your breathing pattern while taking your pulse.

As if by magic or forethought, today's new exercise is called the "Pulse". It can be used for many different exercises but today we will concentrate on the abdominals. I will show you two variations to add to your program.

FBI Pulse #1.

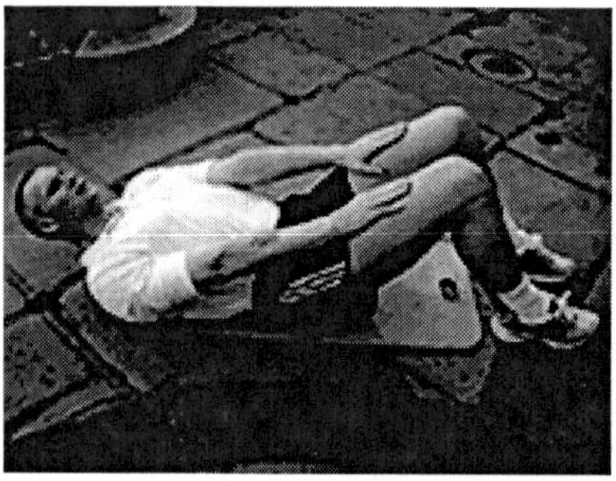

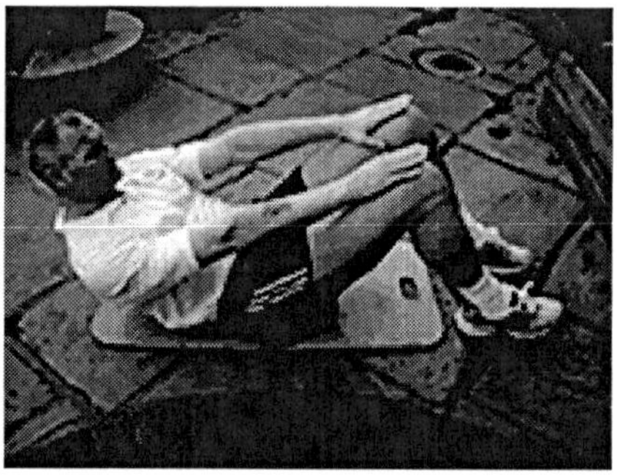

1. First you need to put your stomach muscles under tension.
2. Lie down with your back on your mat.
3. Place your hands on your thighs.
4. Tense your stomach muscles and lift your shoulders off the ground.
5. Keeping the tension in your abdominal muscles reach up to your knees and pulse up and down for the required reps.

FBI Pulse #2.

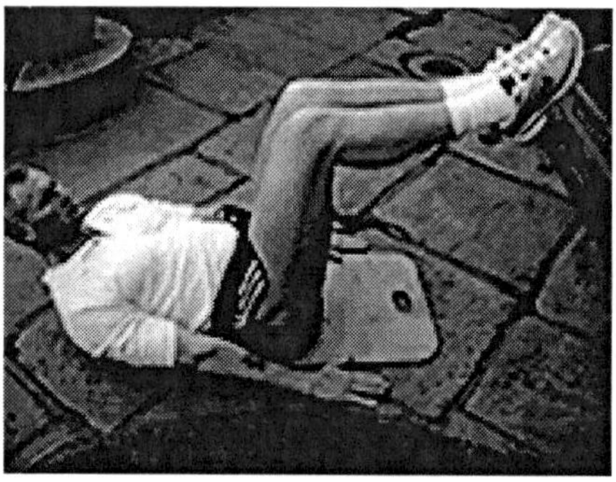

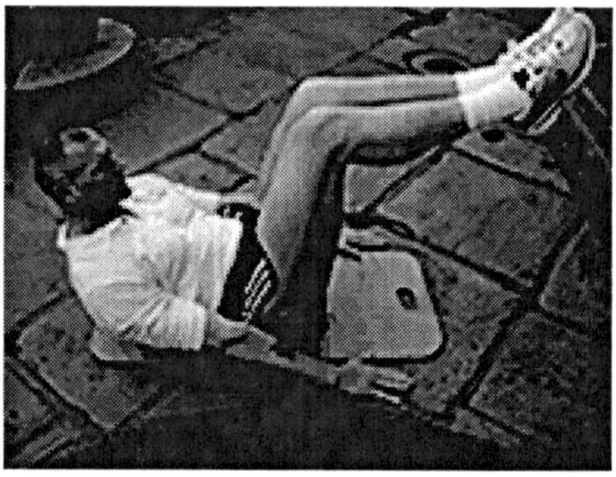

1. The second "pulse" we are going to do is to raise your legs so that your hips and knees are at 90 degrees.
2. Place your hands alongside your body.
3. Reach downwards, keeping your legs still and your hands close to the floor.
4. Pulse for the required number of reps.

COME ON!

- Add “Pulses” to your resistance routine session 2 for 3 sets of 10 reps each.
- Carry out the resistance session 2.

You must be getting stronger by the day.

#66. SIMPLE SUGARS

We talked about the complex carbohydrate the other day, well at the other end of the scale are the simple sugars. Sugar comes in a variety of forms, the most common being “Sucrose”. This is the name given to the white sugar, which is added to tea and coffee or used in baking. Sucrose is a disaccharide made up from Glucose and Fructose (fruit sugar).

Food labels often indicate the presence of other sugars. These include: Glucose, Glucose Syrup, Fructose, Maltose, Honey, Molasses, Dextrose, Corn Syrup and Cane Sugar.

These sugars provide energy, i.e. calories and nothing else. That is why they are referred to as “anti-nutrients”. From a nutritional point of view all sugars are the same. The amount of minerals and vitamins in honey and brown sugars are so minimal that you would have to eat vast quantities of them to get a reasonable amount.

Sugars are also found naturally in foods. Fruit juices and dried fruits, in particular, contain quite a large amount of fructose. The difference here is that the sugars in natural foods do come wrapped up with minerals, vitamins, fibre and starch. Natural sugars need not be limited.

As sugar is a concentrated form of energy it can contribute to the problem of being overweight. This in itself can be associated with other health problems such as heart disease, high blood pressure, diabetes, arthritis to name a few. I’m not saying that sugar is the sole cause of being overweight, but it is easier to eat sweet sugary foods. Lots of snacks are high in sugar and we tend to eat them in addition to our normal diet. Most people can also find room for a sweet even after a full satisfying healthy meal.

As I’ve said before sugar is an “anti-nutrient” containing no vitamins or minerals, yet in order for the body to make use of the sugar it needs the B complex vitamins, magnesium and phosphorous. The body therefore robs itself of existing stores of these nutrients creating nutritional deficiencies.

Have I put you off sugar yet? Well, it's not my intention. Just be aware of how much you're taking in and if you get the opportunity, try to cut down gradually the added sugars in your diet.

How much sugar is in some popular food/drinks?	teaspoons
60 grams Cornflakes	1
50 gram Milk Chocolate bar	5.5
220 grams Canned Peaches in Juice	5
1 Chocolate Digestive Biscuit	1
1 Pint of Beer	2.5
60 grams Sugar Coated Puffs	6
50 grams Wine Gums	11
220 grams Canned Peaches in Syrup	10
1 Plain Digestive	0.5
Large Cola	20

(Total sugar content may vary, depending on the brand)

COME ON!

- A rest day from exercise today.
- Back to the cupboards and food diary again though.
- See where you can cut down on some of the added sugar in your diet.
- Make the adjustments gradually, so that your palate gets used to the gradual decline in added sugar.

#67. PUTTING THE BEANS BACK IN YOUR LIFE

Beans belong to the leguminous family of crops. Simplistically legumes are the foods that come from pods, for example beans, peas and lentils.

The importance of legumes in human diet is well established particularly due to their high nutritional value, long shelf-life, and relatively low cost. Soaking dried beans for a couple of hours brings them back to life, activating enzymes, proteins, minerals and vitamins. They include white beans, black beans, kidney beans, pinto beans, red beans, black-eyed peas, soy beans, lentils, and chick peas.

Beans can be eaten raw (except kidney beans), sprouted or cooked, ground into flour, curdled into tofu, fermented into soya sauce, tempi and miso. They are excellent in chillies, soups and salads. Beans are high in iron and packed with protein. They are also a rich source of thiamin, riboflavin, niacin, potassium, phosphorus and an excellent source of fibre and complex carbohydrates. They are low in sodium and saturated fats.

Beans unfortunately have an unhappy reputation of creating an embarrassing by-product of smelly gas. This gas, which consists mainly of nitrogen and carbon dioxide, is the by-product of bacteria in the intestine breaking down the complex carbohydrates in the beans. I'm sure explaining this will in fact excuse you in anybody's company, or maybe not.

COME ON!

- Cardio session today.
- Get them trainers on and break some records.
- Plot your progress as always and put the beans back in your life.

#68. THICK AS A PLANK

Ever wanted an exercise to do at home that doesn't even seem like hard work? Well this is it. I did say though, it doesn't seem like hard work, but believe me it is. It works all your inner core muscles as you work them iso-metrically. That means that the exercise does not change the length of your working muscles. A static exercise. The exercise in question is called the "Prone Plank".

A plank is strong straight and rigid. The perfect description for such a good strength exercise. It is an excellent exercise for strengthening your core muscles. Strong core muscles are essential for maintaining a strong back.

It is performed using just your body weight and requires no equipment. You may want to rest your forearms on something with a bit of "give" in it though.

FBI Prone Plank

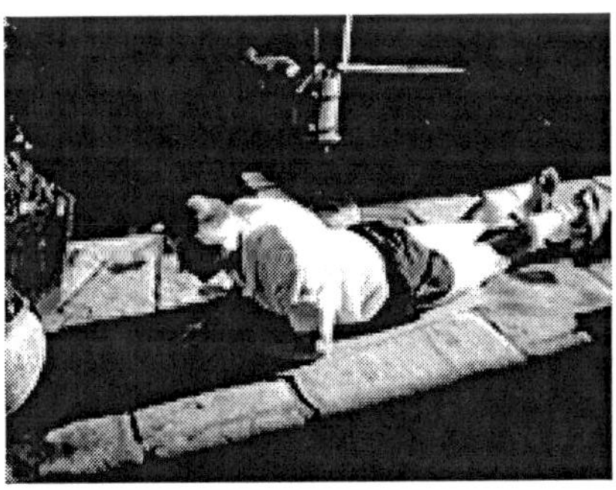

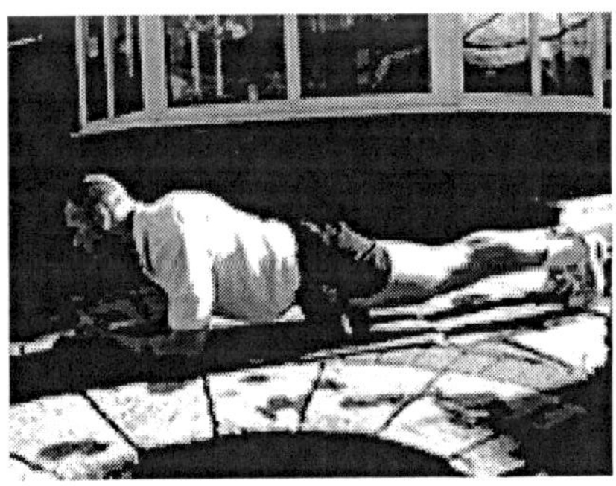

1. Lie face down (prone position) resting on your forearms and your toes.
2. Then simply lift your midriff off the floor so that your body is completely straight.
3. Hold that position for as long as you can.
4. Record how long you can hold the position each time you do the exercise so you can see your improvements.

While we are talking of planks, we may as well turn ourselves over and carry out the opposite exercise, which is called the "Supine Plank".

FBI Supine Plank

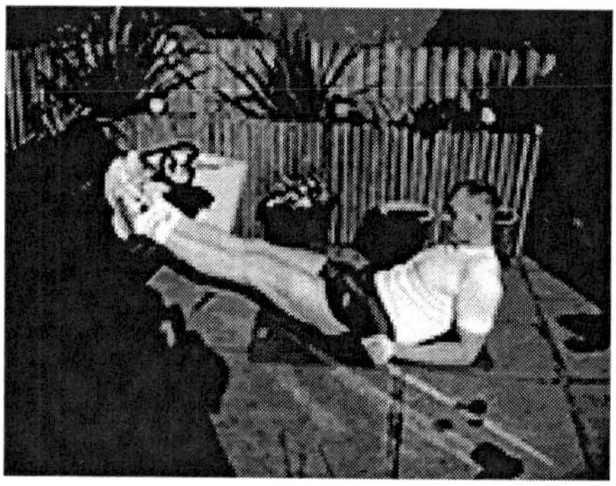

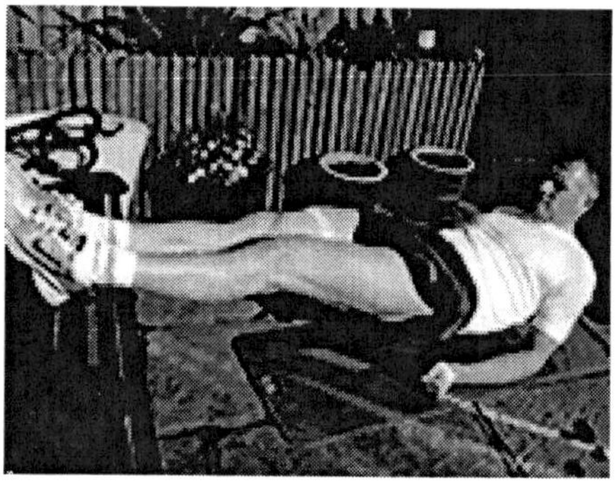

1. Place your heals on a step and rest back onto your forearms.
2. Raise your hips so that your body is in a straight line.
3. Hold the position for as long as you can, making improvements each time you do it.

COME ON!

- Add these exercises to your resistance workout session 1
- Perform 1 x fatigue for each plank.
- Carry out the entire session.

#69. PROTEINS

Proteins are one of the essential food ingredients. They are made up of "Amino Acids" of which there are 20, 8 being essential and 12 being non-essential. They are described as essential if they cannot be formed by the body naturally. Therefore non-essential can be formed by the body.

The role of proteins in the body is split into two major parts:

1. Structural - These are found in muscle, bone, connective tissue and cell walls.
2. Functional - These are found in the hormones, digestive enzymes, anti bodies and neurotransmitters.

Because protein is responsible for the building of muscle it is often assumed and quite wrongly I might add that the more protein you take, the more muscle you will build. Hence all the protein shakes directed at bodybuilders etc. Your body can only utilise a certain amount of protein before turning the remainder into fat deposits. This amount is based on a number of factors:

- Your body size
- Your rate of growth
- The presence or absence of disease
- Your exercise load

We are going to concentrate on two of the factors as they are the variables in our sphere of influence. Your body size (ie weight) and your exercise load.

First we need to know how much protein is recommended. The minimum requirement is 1 gram per 1kg of bodyweight. This figure comes from The National Research Council. This amount is suitable for sedentary people who do not take any exercise and has a non-strenuous job. Not us then. So what are the guidelines for protein intake?

We briefly looked at this on day #9 but now we know a bit more about nutrition we can go a bit deeper.

- **Sedentary person** = 1 gram of protein per 1kg of body weight.
- **Person training hard 3 times a week** = 1.2 - 1.5 grams of protein per 1kg of bodyweight.
- **Athlete doing hard training at least 5 times a week** = 1.5 - 2 grams of protein per 1kg of bodyweight.
- **Athlete involved in heavy resistance sessions 5 times or more a week** = 2 - 2.5 grams of protein per 1kg of bodyweight.

As this is a complicated subject I will talk about complete and incomplete proteins tomorrow when you have digested (pun definitely intended) this information.

COME ON!

- Time to weigh yourself and re-evaluate your protein intake.
- Using the method shown in day #9, make the necessary changes to your calorie requirements for your food diary.
- There should be a difference in your requirements now compared to what you required at the start of the course. This difference will depend on whether you've been losing weight or building your body.

Remember, you are still in control of your destiny. Keep up the good work.

#70. COMPLETE & INCOMPLETE PROTEINS

Proteins are described as being either complete or incomplete.

Complete proteins contain sufficient amounts of all the essential amino acids. Examples of a complete protein food are meat, fish, eggs and dairy products.

Incomplete proteins contain insufficient amounts of the essential amino acids. Nearly all vegetable proteins are incomplete apart from soya products. Therefore vegetarian diets need to be carefully balanced to ensure that all the essential amino acids are taken on board.

Examples of good combinations are:

- Legumes with grains or nuts.
- Milk with grains or nuts or potato or legumes.
- Fresh vegetables with sesame seeds or brazil nuts or rice, or millet or mushrooms.

As you can see, the key to this again is variety. It's back to eating a rainbow and making the food as varied as you can. Experiment with your fresh salads with nuts etc.

COME ON!

- It's your cardio day today.
- 45 minutes of exercise that should have you nicely out of breath.
- Don't forget to stretch the muscles properly when you've finished.
- Record your distance/skips etc to see your progress.

Good work!

#71. SHOULDER THE BURDEN

Your shoulder joints are very flexible, but that flexibility comes with a price. The joint itself is a ball and socket type joint, but unlike the hip joint this has a shallow ball for the socket to fit into. This makes the shoulder joint relatively unstable. In order to stabilise the joint to maintain it's normal function, it requires a lot of muscular control. We have already got exercises in our routine for the front and sides of the shoulder, so today we are looking at developing the rear Deltoids and the Rhomboids (back of the shoulder). It is a lesser-done exercise and often neglected in many a workout but not for us.

The exercise is called "Reverse Flyes".

As the name implies, reverse flyes are a reverse movement of the more commonly performed chest flyes that we looked at on day #62. These can be done using a bench in the gym or freestanding as shown in the photos.

FBI Reverse Flye

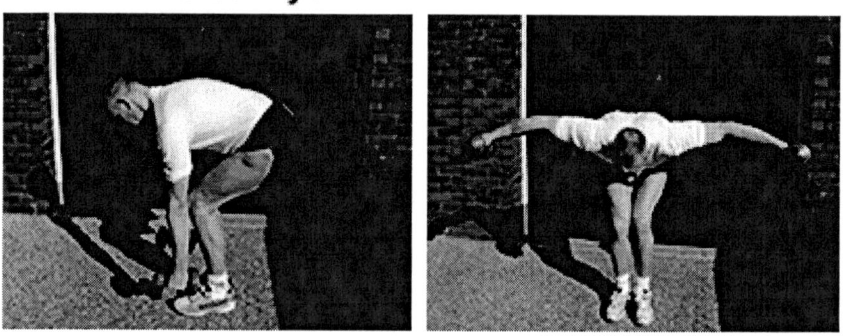

1. Bend the knees and the waist at the hips to get your upper body parallel to the floor.
2. Hold a dumbbell in each hand with your palms facing each other with your arms perpendicular to your body.
3. Keeping the arms slightly bent (soft elbows), raise the dumbbells smoothly out and up to the sides in an arc. Lift

the dumbbells as high as you can in that plane making sure that you don't stray from the perpendicular.
4. Keep your head and torso still and maintain the slight angle at your elbows.
5. Pause for a second at the top of the movement while trying to squeeze your shoulder blades together and downwards.
6. Maintain a slight abdominal contraction to stabilise the pelvis throughout the exercise.
7. Lower your arms back down under control to the start position ready for another rep. That is one rep completed.

As this is an isolation exercise it is best performed after a compound exercise such as the Shoulder Press as shown on day #29.

COME ON!

- Add the reverse flyes to your resistance session 1 for 2 sets of 10 at first (2 x 10)
- Increase your plank exercise to 3 x fatigue now that you are used to the exercise.
- Carry out your entire session 1.

Feeling stronger and looking better by the day, well done.

#72. CHOLESTEROL

Cholesterol is one of those words frequently mentioned but rarely understood. Many people are trying to cut down their cholesterol without really knowing what it is and what function it has within the body. This is the end of all that.

What is Cholesterol? The word cholesterol is a combination of two words, "chole", that means "bile" and "sterol", which means "steroid". Cholesterol is a fatty substance found in all cell membranes. The nervous system contains about 40% of all the cholesterol in the body.

Why do we need cholesterol?

- It maintains the integrity and health of all cell membranes.
- It is involved in the synthesis of sex hormones.
- It is a component of the adrenal cortico-steroids. This is the substance that helps to prepare the body for "freeze, fight or flight" responses to stressful situations. Therefore stress produces cholesterol.
- It is needed for the synthesis of your bile salts.
- It activates the synthesis of vitamin D to get calcium into the blood.
- It helps the kidneys regulate your body's water balance. A cholesterol deficiency can lead to abnormal water retention, which in turn can lead to high blood pressure.

As you can see, cholesterol is important for the correct functioning of the body. We make the required amounts needed for our body. As we take in cholesterol through foods, the body makes adjustments to this level. Cholesterol balance is altered by saturated fat, cholesterol in the diet and hereditary factors. However, an excess of cholesterol in the bile can lead to gallstones and excess in the blood can become deposited on the artery walls leading to "furring" (atheroma) that can then lead on to coronary heart disease (CHD).

Cholesterol is transported around the body as lipoproteins (Fat proteins). They are carried in the blood with proteins in structures very similar to the sweets M&M's or Smarties in the UK. A soft fatty core with a protein shell.

There are four main types of lipoproteins that have slightly different structures and functions within the body. These are:

1. **Chylomicrons (a triglyceride)** - Rich particles formed in the intestine from dietary fats.
2. **VLDL (very low density lipoprotein)** - These transport the triglycerides from the liver to the tissues where it is easily broken down and the cholesterol used.
3. **LDL (low density lipoproteins)** - These transport the cholesterol from the liver to the tissues, where it is broken down less easily than the VLDL's and used for cell membrane metabolism and hormone production etc. Excess levels contribute to the formation of fatty deposits in the blood vessels i.e. atheroma.
4. **HDL (high density lipoprotein)** - These are formed in the tissues from excess LDL's and Chylomicrons. High levels are not associated with atheroma or coronary heart disease. HDL's act as scavengers by removing cholesterol from the blood before it can enter the arterial wall, and return it to the liver.

So as you can see, cholesterol is not as straightforward as it first appears. We need to increase your HDL's and decrease the harmful LDL's. Tomorrow we'll look at some measures that will help you to achieve this.

COME ON!

- A lot of theory today so it is a rest day from exercise.
- Find out where you can get your cholesterol tested. Most good gyms have the equipment to do this.

Take it easy.

#73. INCREASE YOUR HDL'S

Dietary cholesterol only comes from food of animal origin. Foods that are high in dietary cholesterol are egg yolk, cream, full fat milk, cheddar cheese, liver, kidneys and prawns. However, most of the cholesterol in the body does not come from the diet, it is manufactured by body tissues, particularly the liver. A high intake of saturated fat in the diet increases the synthesis of cholesterol in the liver. This happens to varying extents depending on the susceptibility of the individual. This could be a family history of hyper cholesterolaemia.

I have not mentioned what is a high level and what isn't. Different countries have different measurements and methods of recording the results. Some institutions use a standard figure whereas others use a formula based on your blood quantity. Wherever you have the test, they will tell you whether the reading is considered high or not. If the figure is high, you might want to establish whether your cholesterol is high in LDL's or HDL's.

So what can we do to improve the cholesterol in our body? We need to reduce the LDL's and increase our HDL's. Some activities raise your total cholesterol, while others either increase or reduce the individual parts.

- **Increases healthy HDL's** - Exercise, maintaining a healthy weight and the use of monounsaturated fats.
- **Reduces harmful LDL's** Soluble fibre, omega 3 fish oil and substituting saturated fats with monounsaturated fats.
- **Reduces total cholesterol** - Exercise and the use of polyunsaturated fats.
- **Increases total cholesterol** - Stress, excess use of alcohol.
- **Reduces healthy HDL's** - Smoking.
- **Increases harmful LDL's** - Smoking (possible), high dietary saturated fats intake.

Some of the activities give you a double whammy effect by increasing the good and reducing the bad. Exercise is one of these. What a shock eh?

COME ON!

- It is a cardio day today.
- Think of your cholesterol levels as you train your cardio vascular system.
- Record your results as always and see the improvements.

#74. GET THE RIGHT KIT

It is very important to have the right kit when you are training. Now I'm not talking about designer labels here. On the contrary, any old loose fitting clothing will do if you're exercising just so long as you're comfortable.

The kind of kit I'm talking about are the essentials.

Training shoes are important items of kit as you only have one pair of feet so you have to look after them. Again, I'm not talking about top of the range shoes here. Go for a comfortable pair that is designed for the type of training that you are doing. For the purpose of this course it would be sufficient to be using a "cross-trainer". This is one step down from your fully-fledged "running" shoe. I would recommend specialised running shoes if you were to start to take your running more seriously. A definite if a marathon is being considered.

Protective equipment is also a must for you. If you're cycling it is recommended that you get a proper fitting cycle helmet. If you're into boxing or any other martial arts, then a gum shield is required so that you can smile with confidence when you achieve your goals. For the ladies (especially the well endowed ones) a correctly fitting sports (supportive) bra is a must.

Today's new resistance exercise is called the "Single Arm Row". Typically this is done by leaning forward, so that the upper body is both supported and nearly parallel to the floor, and raising your weight (dumbbell) from the floor vertically up towards the torso using a rowing type movement. Unlike a number of back exercises, each side of the back is worked independently.

A good range of muscles are used in this exercise. The Latissimus Dorsi (upper back and side) is the dominant muscle being exercised. Assisting in this exercise is the Rear Deltoids, Biceps, middle fibres of the Trapezius muscles and the Rhomboids. As you can see a lot of muscles are involved.

You can use a bench for this exercise but I will show you how to do this with no extra kit.

FBI Single Arm Row

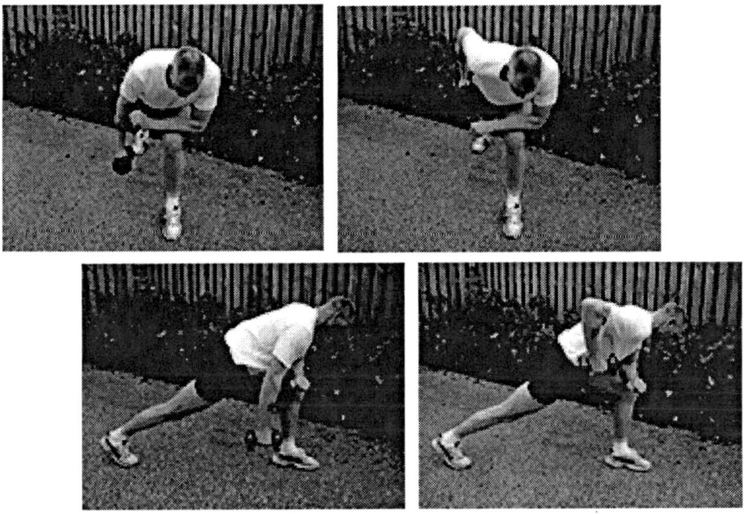

1. Take an exaggerated step forward with your left leg.
2. Lean forward supporting the weight of your upper body with your left forearm on your thigh.
3. Ensure that your shoulders are parallel to the floor throughout the exercise and that the torso does not twist, as it will raise one of your shoulders. Usual causes for this are looking at the weight as you lift it or trying to lift a weight that is too heavy for you.
4. Before you lift the weight with your right hand. Let the weight hang freely at first, then begin to lift the weight vertically (in a straight line) by bending your right elbow until the weight reaches the side of your chest.
5. Concentrate on bringing your shoulder blades together throughout the lift.
6. Like all the previous resistance exercises, we breathe out when we "do the work". On this exercise it is when we lift the weight.
7. Pause for a second when the weight is at the top of the movement before returning the weight under control to the floor. That is one rep completed.
8. Do the recommended amount of reps before changing over sides.

COME ON!

- Add your "Single Arm Row" to session 2 for 2 x 10.
- Alter your "Step-overs" to 3 x 15 (each leg).
- Carry out the full session 2.

#75. EATING DISORDERS

Many people have some sort of eating disorder. Some are open about it and some hide it from their partners, family and friends (some better than others). So what is an eating disorder? Before we define the disorder, it's necessary to know what we mean by "normal" eating.

Normal eating involves regular meals and snacks to sustain the body throughout its working day. The body recognises signals of hunger and acknowledges being satisfied. Food, body image and our weight will occupy approximately 10% of our total daily thoughts.

A disordered eating pattern occurs when we consistently eat more or less than what the body requires. Most of the day will be consumed with thoughts of food and calories. The result of eating is guilt, depression, anger and shame.

There are countless reasons for eating disorders from emotional to physical problems and each case must be tackled separately. Research does show that anyone can develop an eating disorder although your genetic make up could make you more predisposed. As well as the biological aspect, external influences also have a large and adverse contribution. It could develop from a comment from a family member or the result of a traumatic event. Bullying, emotional, physical or sexual abuse or the loss of a loved one, illness and divorce are other contributing factors.

The media portrays the images of what is society's acceptable "body shape" as do most of the glamour magazines that are found on the shelves of the newsagents. In a world that is obsessed with body image it is no surprise that some individuals will go to incredible, drastic and often fatal lengths to attain the "perfect body". This course is hopefully demonstrating that the results you are seeking can be reached following sensible and sustainable methods.

The most common eating disorder is **Bulimia Nervosa**. This is a never-ending cycle of binge eating followed by a purging. The purging can consist of different methods like vomiting, laxatives, diuretics, diet pills etc. Each one having their own differing results.

Bulimia is the most difficult eating disorder to recognise, as sufferers may appear to eat normally.

Anorexia Nervosa is most common among young girls between 13 and 17 as they fight the natural development of their body. Anorexics are obsessed with thinness and will intentionally starve themselves as they have an irrational fear of calories and weight gain. Regardless of how underweight they are, they will see themselves to be fat and avoid eating at all costs in their quest to lose weight. They may exercise excessively and/or use the same methods as a bulimic. Stepping on the scales ten times a day is not uncommon, or spending an abnormal time in front of a mirror, not for vanity, but in despair over the distorted image that is before them. Most anorexics will avoid seeking help as they know that this will end up in them having to eat. The weight loss makes individuals more susceptible to conditions such as osteoporosis, heart and kidney problems. For female sufferers the drop in body weight and the loss of essential fats will result in disrupted menstrual cycles leaving fertility problems.

A **"Compulsive Overeater"** will suffer uncontrollable urges to eat resulting in significant weight gain. Food will be used to block out any negative emotion or situation that they come across. It is similar to what we call "comfort eating" but on a greater scale. They will often eat alone, however if they are in company they will often only eat a small amount to hide their problem. Many overeaters will withdraw from any social activity, as they feel so self-conscious about their weight. This isolation leads to depression, low esteem and feelings of inadequacy, fuelling the need to binge even more. The bigger the weight gain, the increased effort to lose it by dieting. The resulting failure of the diet will result in more negative feelings starting the cycle off again.

All bad news? Well not quite. Treatments of all eating disorders require nutritional rehabilitation and psychological help. Learning to like what you've hated for so long is not an easy task by any means, but it isn't impossible. The first thing that is required is the will of the individual. Without this, any action is doomed to failure. There are many help groups in the world set up by people who have been through it themselves and have found strategies that combat the various illnesses.

I myself use the knowledge of the body and what it needs to survive healthily in order to help my clients. I use education, like this course, in general to show that good fuel and good exercise can give the person the healthy body they generally require. It is a difficult fight but I fight irrationality with fact. Not a bad weapon to have on your side.

Most of today's lesson might seem irrelevant to a lot of you but if it helps just one person out there, then I think it has been well worth the effort. It may help you to understand what other people go through or just encourage you to read further into this massive subject.

Phew! Have a rest today.

#76. ENJOY YOUR TRAINING

Life is too short to be doing things in life that we don't enjoy. Likewise, you must enjoy the training that you are doing. If you are not enjoying it you might not keep it up. I don't know many people that will keep on doing something on a regular basis that is a real chore. Exercise is no different in this instance. So how do we ensure that you are enjoying it? Well I can't from here and that's a fact. But what I can offer is some sound advice.

Motivation is often borne out of achievement. If you are making good progress in the healthy lifestyle bit and your exercise capability has improved, you will no doubt be very pleased with yourself. When we get good at things we tend to enjoy them more. So everything spirals, the more you enjoy it, the more passion you put into your training and the more passion you put in, the better the results and so on.

Variety helps to keep the fun factor going. That's why I try and do something different every time I train. Not only does it prevent boredom, it also works slightly different muscles. This ensures that your body does not get out of balance by over-training one specific set of muscles.

COME ON!

- It is your cardio day today.
- Take a look at what you haven't done for a while. Are you getting into a routine and ignoring other activities?
- Today could be the day that you change that trend.
- Make a special effort today to do something different.
- Record your results as always. Does it make for good reading? I bet it does.

Well done!

#77. KEEP YOUR JACKET ON

Ever had jacket potatoes? The answer is probably yes. Well, some people actually have these and then throw away the most nutritious part. The skin. Just under the skin of vegetables, the majority of the goodness is found and when peeled is subsequently lost.

I have not peeled a vegetable for years and years, which not only is it giving me that extra goodness, it also saves me time when preparing meals. It's not just potatoes, but also carrots, swede, turnips, parsnips etc. In fact anything that people generally peel, I don't. I do make sure though that I thoroughly wash the vegetables. It's not only the goodness and time you're saving. What about the money? There's more edible food for your money too. Talk about a "win-win" situation.

The same is said for all the fruits that have edible skins. Washed thoroughly, there's more to eat if you don't peel them.

The resistance sessions are now complete so we will be looking at different types of resistance training in the up and coming resistance days. You are still doing the "muscle build" program to increase your lean muscle tissue. I generally keep people on this type of training for 6 to 8 weeks before I change to a strength program. As we have not completed a full 6 weeks on most of the exercises, we will remain on this for the duration of the course.

COME ON!

- Resistance session 1 today.
- Increase your "Reverse Flyes" to 3 x 8-12

I bet your press-ups have increased quite a bit since the start. Does it make you feel good? It should do.

#78. GREEN IS ALSO FOR JEALOUSY

This is where you have to be careful. There are some people out there that will be pleased if you fail in this latest quest to become fit and healthy. I know you will find this one hard to believe but some people will actually resent you having the success that you are striving for. They will go to extra-ordinary efforts to try and make you relapse into unhealthy ways.

Why, you might ask? This could be for numerous reasons. Maybe they have been trying for years too, to lose the weight or get fitter generally. You are now streets ahead of them and they just know that they cannot catch you up. Maybe your change in lifestyle has made you a more confident and out going person. Your spouse might not like the thought of this "new person" with high self-esteem going out. People's reactions change when you change, so just be aware of the new circumstances that you might find yourself in.

The tricks they might use are:

- Taking in cakes and biscuits into work. They could be left out where you might be passing or offered to you in a way that suggests, "go on, one won't hurt" As we know, one generally leads to lots. If they are part of your controlled eating plan, then by all means enjoy them. Remember, life is all about enjoyment.
- A few drinks and nibbles. Again, don't be obliged to eat them because they're there. Even worse is the suggestion that you have a "take away" after the drinks. I'm pretty sure that you'd have already had your meals for the day, so an extra one would all be extra calories.
- People saying, "oh you don't need to lose any more weight, you look fine the way you are". Now is that fine for them or fine for you? Remember, you decide. It is your training plan and your life.

On this note though, don't become paranoid, just be aware. Don't let others influence your eating or drinking patterns. You have found a way that works comfortably for you and is sustainable. Stick with it and see the results in the coming weeks.

COME ON!

- Rest day today. A chance therefore to catch up on any parts that you have not done.
- Keep it going and feel proud of your achievements so far.

Well done, see you tomorrow.

#79. LEARN TO DANCE

As today is a cardio day, there is a healthy alternative that seems like too much fun to be "good for you". That alternative is "Dancing". We don't need to join a dance class or leave the comfort of your own home. Just pop on your favourite cd and dance away.

Sounds simple doesn't it? Well if you think of it, it is. High-powered music that you can lose yourself in can burn tons of energy and get the sweat pouring from you in minutes. You will get the same benefits in the cardio-vascular department if you're puffing away as you would in your normal cardio session.

For the more adventurous, there are many dance classes about these days from "Salsa" to "Line-Dancing". The beauty of dancing is that you don't even realise that you are working out. Going back a couple of days, if you enjoy what you are doing, you will do it more.

The average hourly calorie expenditure for the cardio-vascular exercise in our program so far is roughly

Exercise (1 hr)	Women (calories)	Men (calories)
Walking moderate	168	224
Jogging	444	592
Running	692	900
Rowing	600	800
Cycling (moderate)	192	256
Cycling (hard)	507	660
Skipping	476	635
Dancing (Ballroom)	264	352

As you can see, even dancing will get those calories shifted, certainly make you lighter on your feet and improve your co-ordination. Co-ordination is linked with balance and as we get older, that is one thing that seems to diminish. Great benefits from just having fun eh? The only thing is that dancing is not really measurable, so how do you know you're getting better? Just ask your partner; they'll soon tell you.

COME ON!

- Cardio day today. Dancing or running? Straddles or Skipping? Or maybe Cycling or Rowing.
- Now don't say you're bored.
- Work hard and get a good sweat on.

Go on and dance!

#80. STRENGTH & POWER TRAINING

Our 3 sets of exercises are sufficient for beginners to resistance training, but what about if you want to carry on and build more muscle and increase strength further. Well you will continue to progress doing 3 sets but there are further steps that you could take. Unless you have an extensive range of equipment available to you, you might need to enter a gym for this progression. Don't worry though you are more than capable of holding your own in these places. Just don't pick up bad habits.

We have concentrated on building lean muscle so far. This is called "Hypertrophy", the greater the number of muscle fibres fatigued, the greater the hypertrophy. The key being to choose a rep range and weight that will recruit as many fibres as possible. An 8 to 12 rep range has been seen to be the most efficient. This would be carried out anywhere from 3 to 20 sets per muscle groups (depends on whether you're working big muscle groups, which would be a larger number, or smaller muscle groups, which would be a smaller number). Obviously the amount you do would depend on the time you have available and how intense you are training. The rest period is between 30 and 90 seconds between sets.

So where do we go from here? Now that we have built some new muscle, we must start to put some strength into it. As a general rule, high resistance and lower reps is the best method for increasing muscular strength. The rep range for the development of strength is between 3 and 8. This would be carried out anywhere from 3 to 10 sets per muscle groups. Again the amount you do would depend on the time you have available and how intense you are training. The rest period is between 2 and 5 minutes between sets. Good recovery is required for strength training.

The next step is to put power into the muscles. Power is the improvement of speed of contraction against resistance rather than maximum strength itself. As the speed of contraction increases, the amount of force developed decreases. To increase your power, high loads, 90% of your 1RM (1 repetition of your maximum lift - the heaviest weight you can lift only once) are used in an explosive manner. Lighter weights could be used but because of the high speeds involved you would have to let go of the weight to prevent joint injury. Medicine balls (weighted balls) are ideal if you do not have sufficient weight to lift. You would perform anywhere from 3 to 10 sets per muscle groups. Yet again the amount you do would depend on the time you have available and how intense you are training. The rest period is between 2 and 5 minutes between sets.

Remember when you are doing the exercises to failure you must stick to the strictest form throughout your exercise. A loss of form is an indication of a fully fatigued muscle. The best example of this is when performing your "shoulder press" exercise, if you started to arch your back to lift a few more repetitions you are actually trying to recruit your chest muscles to help your shoulders. Be aware of your form at all times.

COME ON!

- It is your resistance session number 2 today.
- Concentrate on your good form.

#81. GET A PERSONAL TRAINER

Now I know you probably don't need a Personal Trainer because you've been motivated enough to come this far. So why am I saying this? It could be self-preservation of my profession. A nice thought, but no. A personal trainer can keep that motivation and direction going if you ever start to drift. Hopefully this will not be the case but there's no harm in setting out a plan beforehand.

What can a Personal Trainer do for you? After finding out about your likes, dislikes, strengths, weaknesses and goals, he will assess your current level of fitness and suggest the best way forward to achieve your goals. He will devise a fitness programme to specifically target your needs. You already have a great basic programme but if you are training for a specific sport or event (e.g. a Marathon) he will adjust your training plan accordingly to suit your needs.

Is there a typical session? Well not with me. Everything revolves around you and your requirements. If you don't like running, then we would do something else to suit you. The weather and time available will also determine what happens on the day. The presence of niggles or injuries may decide what you can do and can't do. The main emphasis is creating a fun environment in which to train effectively in. So if I'm doing that, I imagine they all are.

How often would I need one? This would depend on how motivated you remain. I train people from 3 times a week to once a month. If you are highly motivated, you may never need one other than to get a specific program. If you're well motivated with a few slips, then it might be the "once a month" kick up the backside that is sufficient to keep you on track. Everyone is different and who am I to tell you how to spend your money. I personally hope that you never need help again, but just in case.

COME ON!

- Another well earned rest day.
- Find out who the Personal Trainers are in your area.

#82. STRETCHING THE LIMITS

Stretching is carried out to increase our flexibility. Many active participants often overlook it but overlook it at your peril. Flexibility can vary dramatically from one person to the next. The two extremes are those who appear to be "double jointed", an erroneous title given to someone who has a high degree of flexibility or hyper-mobility. Gymnasts and dancers might fall into this category. The other is a significant lack of flexibility resulting in impaired or painful performance. There is no one test to give a true indication of your flexibility, as it is specific to each joint in the body.

Certain sports are responsible for a reduction in muscle flexibility. This is because your muscles are not worked through their full range. Jogging, football, cycling, boxing to name but a few of the sports. Muscle shortening can also result from poor posture or when a body part is immobilised for a period of time. An imbalance of muscle is also a problem for example where the quadriceps are trained but the hamstrings are not. The best example of this is where a lady wears high heels all the time and the calf muscles, Achilles tendon are not stretched even when walking.

The benefits of a regular flexibility programme are:

- **Reduced risk of injury.** Stretching improves the range of movement of a muscle, which will then allow greater movement of a joint when stretched to its limit.
- Increasing and encouraging full range of movement across a joint enables **greater speed and power** to be achieved. Examples of this are the javelin and the throwing of a ball.
- **Decreased muscle stiffness after exercise.** Stretching after your session can diminish muscle tightening and prevent stiffness developing by assisting in venous return. This disperses the lactic acid and waste products from the muscles, which cause the stiffness.
- **In rehabilitation from injury**, stretching is essential in stretching out the fibrous tissue (scar tissue) before it

hardens. Scar tissue is not flexible and will therefore always be a weak point in a muscle if left to develop.

- **Relaxation, Stress Reduction and Improved Body Awareness.** Most stretch classes are performed lying on the floor for stability purposes. You are encouraged to breathe slowly and to stretch one muscle group at a time.

Some of the factors that affect our flexibility are:

- **Age.** We all know that babies bounce (but don't try this at home). Babies and infants are very flexible; you only have to see them with their foot wedged in their own mouth to confirm this.
- **Sex.** Females are generally more flexible than males. The reason is not fully understood but may well be due to the different activities that they do when they are young. Females however, during pregnancy and in the post-natal period produce a hormone "relaxin" to assist in childbirth giving greater flexibility. This greater flexibility is not confined to the pelvic area so caution must be observed so that they don't overstretch the joints during this period.
- **Temperature.** An increase in temperature can increase the flexibility of a muscle. Conversely, cold temperatures can decrease the flexibility by as much as 20%.
- **Heredity.** Some people are born with an inherited characteristic of hyper-mobility. There can be risk of dislocation of some joints and therefore strength training round the specific joints would be recommended.
- **Exercise.** Active people tend to be more flexible than sedentary people.
- **Fashion.** Adaptive shortening of the Achilles tendon and calf muscles can occur due to the constant wearing of high heels. If prolonged use is required or desired, ensure that you stretch your calf muscles even more regularly.

Tomorrow I will go into the different types of stretching that you can do.

COME ON!

- Time to stretch your limits with your cardio program.
- Ensure that your mobility and warm-up is still an integral part of your session.
- Cool down properly and record your progress.

#83. TYPES OF STRETCHING

Today we are going to look at the different types of stretching that you can perform.

- **Static** - Static stretching is where the muscle is taken to the end of its normal range and held without bouncing.
- **Ballistic** - This form of stretching involves quick repetitive bouncing actions in order to increase the stretch beyond the muscle's normal range using momentum and bodyweight. It is generally considered unacceptable for the average exerciser. However there are times when this more radical method is used to stretch adhesions and stubborn fibrous tissue in physiotherapy and rehabilitation.
- **Active** - This method uses a contracted muscle or muscle group to stretch the opposing muscle. For example hamstrings actively contract to stretch the quadriceps.
- **Passive** - This is where another body part or external factor is used to facilitate the stretch. For example, lying on your back and stretching your hamstrings by placing the hands behind the knee and pulling back.
- **PNF or Proprioceptor Neuromuscular Facilitation** - PNF involves a static stretch followed by an isometric (static) contraction for about 6 - 10 seconds of a muscle against an immoveable resistance (could be a partner). The muscle is then relaxed and stretched further statically and the action is repeated. The muscles have to be very warm to perform this stretch. It is recommended that you use this type of stretch under the supervision or help of a qualified fitness professional.
- **Dynamic** - This is similar to ballistic stretching, but the movement of the limb is not activated by momentum or external forces but by the use of the body's own musculature. An example of this is the hip flexors will flex the hip in order to stretch the hamstrings.

Now you know why we didn't go deep into stretching earlier on in the course. Static stretching will serve your purpose well at this stage in your training, but you are now aware that there are other more advanced methods kicking around.

The field of flexibility training has only recently attracted the interests of researchers and there is still much to learn on the subject. There is little evidence to prove that stretching during the warm-up phase of your workout will reduce the risk of injury. On the contrary, it is widely believed that minor muscle fibre tears can occur when stretching muscles that are not fully warmed up.

General guidelines for stretching are:

- Breathe calmly and rhythmically. Be patient, concentrate and work smoothly throughout the session.
- Whenever possible, stretch in either a sitting or a lying position for stability.
- Stretch towards the end of each workout as a minimal requirement. The muscles should be very warm and receptive to extension.

COME ON!

- It's your resistance session number 1 today.
- I bet your "plank" exercise is pretty impressive by now.

#84. MINERALS

Minerals are elements that are found in abundance in the earth's crust. As constituents of various enzyme systems in the body, they are vital factors in our well-being and health.

It could be said that minerals are more important than vitamins because vitamins depend on minerals for their absorption. It is therefore important that we become conscious of our mineral intake.

Minerals do not work alone. They work as a team and therefore it is vital that you get all your minerals in your daily diet. Supplementation is not generally needed, as the body cannot store excesses of minerals.

There are two types of minerals, macrominerals and trace minerals sometimes known as trace elements.

Macrominerals - These are needed in larger amounts in the body. The main macrominerals are Calcium (Ca), Magnesium (Mg), Sodium (Na) refer back to day #34 and Potassium (K). They are supplied to the body through plant and animal foods. They have a very important role in metabolism and help to regulate heartbeat, water balance and the functioning of nerves and muscles.

Good sources of macrominerals are:

Calcium Ca	Magnesium Mg	Sodium Na	Potassium K
Milk, Leafy green vegetables	Legumes, Wholegrains	Shellfish, Bacon	Salmon/Tuna, Bananas

The list obviously could go on but I have stuck with just 2 examples of each.

Trace Minerals - These are necessary in smaller amounts. They are Iron, Zinc, Copper, Manganese, Chromium, Iodine, Selenium, Flourine and Molybdenum. They each form less than one hundredth of one percent of the human body. They are however vitally important to health as deficiencies of trace minerals can result in various symptoms, for example, iron deficiency can cause anaemia. Although trace minerals are indispensable to the body, excess is not desirable and can also cause problems. Some trace elements such as Lead, Cadmium, Mercury and Aluminium are highly toxic even in miniscule amounts and should be avoided.

Good sources of trace minerals are:

Iron	Offal meats, vegetables, wholegrains, egg yolk
Copper	Offal meats, seafood
Chromium	Wholegrains, shellfish
Selenium	Seafood, meat
Molybdenum	Wholegrains, legumes
Zinc	Meats, eggs, seafood
Manganese	Wholegrains, black tea
Iodine	Seafood

A rest day today from exercise. Tomorrow we'll take a look at vitamins.

#85. VITAMINS

Vitamins are micro-nutrients found in varying amounts in all natural vegetable and animal foods. Each food has a different concentration of specific vitamins. A few vitamins are made by the body, but most are provided by the food that we eat. There are about 20 vitamins known to be vital to human nutrition.

There is no general formula to determine how much of each vitamin we require, but there are tables that have been drawn up that recommends how much we need to take. Two such tables are:

- **RDAs** - Recommended Daily Allowances - published by the Food and Nutrition Board of the National Research Council of the Academy of Sciences to protect public health.
- **SONAs** - Suggested Optimal Nutrient Allowance - by Dr Emanuel Cheraskin and Ringsdorf from the University of Alabama.

Many food product labels will use the RDAs to tell you how much you are taking. Sometimes this is a percentage figure. Many whole foods contain all the vitamins we need for a healthy life. Remember to "eat a rainbow" as different coloured foods will have different vitamins in it. A simple guideline.

On supplementation, I refer back to day #60 and emphasise that if you get enough vitamins through food, then taking a multi-vitamin for the sake of it could turn into expensive urine.

So what are the main vitamins and what are good sources of food. Well here is a small guide and by no means exhaustive.

Vitamin	Main Uses	Good Food Source
A - Retinol	Vision, skin and mucous membranes, cell growth, reproduction and normal immunity.	Liver, fish liver oils, carrots, dark green leafy vegetables.

B1 - Thiamin	Helps to maintain normal energy metabolism.	Whole grains
B2 - Riboflavin	Helps the mitochondria (your ovens) of your muscle cells to produce energy.	Meats, poultry, fish and dairy produce.
B3 - Niacin	Works in the glycogen energy cycle, the oxidation of fatty acids for energy, and in the tissue respiration.	Meats and fish.
B5 - Pantothenic Acid	Necessary for making of glucose and fatty acids, the main fuels of the body. It is also essential for making steroid hormones and brain neurotransmitters.	Liver, fish, cereals and whole grain bread.
B6 - Pyridoxine	Making of haemoglobin and all new proteins. It is also essential for an enzyme that breaks down muscle glycogen for fuel.	Wheat germ, chicken, fish and eggs.
Folate - Folic Acid	Control amino acid metabolism.	Dark green leafy vegetables, legumes and egg yolk.
B12 - Cyanocobalamin	Essential for all cells, particularly rapid-turnover cells, including red blood cells, the lining of the gastrointestinal tract and	Animal foods.

	bone marrow cells.	
Biotin	Enables the proper use of fat or glucose for fuel, breaks down and subsequently builds up new proteins.	Liver, sardines, egg yolk and soy flour.
C - Ascorbate	Antioxidant.	Fruit and green vegetables.
D - Cholecalciferol	Bone growth and mineral balance.	Milk and dairy. Sunlight allows the body to synthesize vitamin D on the skin.
E - D-alpha-tocopherol	Antioxidant.	Liver, butter, eggs, Fruit, green vegetables, cereals and bread.
K - Phylloquinone	Enables your blood to clot.	Green leafy vegetables.

Again it can be seen that eating a balanced diet will enable the body to obtain the necessary vitamins required for a healthy life.

COME ON!

- It's your cardio day today.
- As usual, work hard and burn those calories.

#86. THE ALTERNATIVE APPROACH

Today we are going to look at some alternative types of resistance training. These can help to keep your training fresh and fun. The alternatives we will look at is "Supersetting", "Pyramids" and "Drop Sets".

Supersetting

This is popular with busy people because it allows a greater volume of work for the same amount of time. Here we alternate exercises between opposing body parts. The advantage here is that the recovery time can be kept to a minimum since for example the chest recovers as the back is worked and vice-versa. This condenses the workout allowing for more sets to be done within a given time frame or just to cut short your time in your gym (wherever that may be). Examples of exercises are Bicep curls - Tricep dips and Press-ups - Pull-ups.

Supersetting is less relevant to strength and power work since time must be allowed for near full recovery between sets to allow your energy stores to replenish.

Pyramids

These can be performed either way to vary your training. This type of training is best done on resistance machines where you can change the weight very quickly. Likewise if you have a good range of preset dumbbells, that would also suffice. The examples are just nominal weights used just for illustration. You would perform your pyramid with weights appropriate to your strength level.

Example 1 - Bench Press

10 reps at 50kg - 8 reps at 60kg - 6 reps at 70kg - 4 reps at 80kg - 2 reps at 90kg - 1 rep at 100kg

3 reps at 85kg - 5 reps at 75kg - 7 reps at 65kg - 9 reps at 55 reps - 11 reps at 45kg.

Example 2 - Bench Press

1 rep at 100kg - 2 reps at 90kg - 4 reps at 80kg - 6 reps at 70kg - 8 reps at 60kg - 10reps at 50kg and then return up to the top again finishing at 1 rep at 100kg.

The weights and reps are your choice to play about with. Have fun with them when you find your training going a bit stale.

Drop Sets

These are also called "stripping" and are used to increase the intensity of the workout. It does this by recruiting and fatiguing a wider range of muscle fibres. It involves completing a set at a given weight then immediately "working to complete failure" with a lighter weight and repeating this 2 or 3 times with progressively lighter weights. This type of workout is more suited to an advanced trainer, so beware, you will feel some muscle soreness afterwards if you've done it right. Remember to stretch properly after these drop sets.

There are many other different types of training schedules that you may come across in magazines. By all means have a play when you need a boost. Any training is better than none. Always remember your main training routine though.

COME ON!

- Resistance session 2 today.
- Alter your "Single Arm Row" to 3 x 8-12

Nearly there, well done so far.

#87. SPECIAL POPULATIONS

I have found that people with medical conditions are often put to one side when it comes to health and fitness. In my experience there are too few places that offer good facilities for people with disabilities. Today we're going to talk about people with various medical conditions and I call them the "Special Populations". There are benefits a plenty for these people as I know from personal experience as many of my private clients belong to this group. If you know anyone who does not train because of a "perceived" belief that exercise is not for them, please refer them to this course. It definitely includes them.

Overview of the benefits of physical activity to identified special populations are as follows:

- **Coronary heart disease (CHD)** - Exercise helps to reverse the established disease and helps to control the risk factors for heart disease. The risk factors are high blood pressure, high cholesterol and obesity.
- **Stroke** - Exercise helps to prevent strokes and it helps to restore function after a stroke.
- **High Blood Pressure** - Exercise serves as a drug free therapy for treating mild to moderate high blood pressure (hypertension). It also helps people who are on medication to reduce their blood pressure leading to a reduction and sometimes a cessation of their medication.
- **Diabetes** - Exercise and diet can improve blood glucose control and thereby prevent or delay some of the serious vascular complications of diabetes. I have worked with individuals who have dramatically cut their medication due to the lowering of their blood sugar levels.
- **Obesity** - Exercise and diet helps people in improving or optimising their bodyfat levels.
- **Arthritis** - Exercise improves the flexibility and joint range of motion. It also increases the endurance and strength of the supporting musculature.

- **Osteoporosis** - Exercise can prevent and reverse bone loss thereby protecting against fractures and general bone degeneration.
- **Asthma** - Exercise provides both physical and mental benefits through improvements to respiratory function.
- **Cancer** - Exercise and diet can decrease the risk of certain cancers like colon and breast cancer.
- **Stress/Depression** - Exercise and diet can reduce depression and anxiety, increases feelings of well-being, improves ability to handle stress and improve self image.
- **Multiple Sclerosis (MS)** - Exercise can reduce the debilitating effects of MS. Balance can be improved and muscle strength can also be dramatically increased.

This list is by no means exhaustive but it gives you some idea of the awaiting benefits that can be had by anybody regardless of their physical ability at present. Remember, we're all human.

COME ON!

- This is the final rest day of your course.
- Have you been using your rest days wisely and indulging in some relaxation therapy? If not, this is the day. Do something different and enjoy.

#88. SELF ESTEEM

Do you love yourself? Do you believe you are a good person? If the answer to these 2 questions is a resounding "Yes", then you have got good self-esteem. If the answer was a yes-ish, then you have a little bit of work to do. If on the other hand there was a "No", oh dear, read on.

Having a high self-esteem means that you believe yourself to be a good person and you love yourself unconditionally. Warts and all by the way. It doesn't mean that you don't make the occasional mistake and that you can't learn anything from anyone. That is arrogance. It means that you have the compassion and humanity to learn from your mistakes, knowing that every mistake gives you an opportunity to improve. Self-esteem is also having the confidence to take risks, to learn new ways and skills, to put new ideas into operation and to accept challenges. It represents a healthy sense of perspective.

Having a high self-esteem is closely related to humility, not to an exaggerated sense of self-importance or of being superior to others. A person with a high self-esteem has a healthy attitude about their faults and doesn't feel a need to deny them.

On the other side of the coin, having a low self-esteem is closely linked to self-hatred and some people actually hate themselves. Sometimes for an action that has happened to them quite some time ago and outside their particular sphere of influence. Most people with low self-esteem suffer from a lack of purpose in their life.

There are ways to increase your self-esteem. Some of the ways are easier than others. That is because some of them dig down deep to our beliefs whether they're right or wrong.

Here are some tips:

- Have a sense of humour - do not take yourself too seriously. You are only human after all.
- Be positive - the world can seem a brighter place if you think your glass is half full instead of half empty.

- See something good in everything and everybody - you may have to look hard, but something good will be there.
- Do not hold grudges - clear the air by all means, but don't let an incident eat away inside you, especially when it's over with.
- Be motivated by your own values - get excited about who you are and what you stand for.
- Be forgiving of yourself - don't beat yourself up for not doing something or straying from your chosen path. This goes for allowing yourself a treat without feeling guilty when you've been working hard.
- Value other people - if you value and accept people for being human, you know that you don't have to act in a particular way to be liked and valued in return. This allows you to be yourself.
- Accept criticism - constructive criticism is not personal so don't take it that way. Listen to it, welcome it and most of all learn from it. Your self-evaluation is more important than someone else's opinion, so take what is useful and throw away the rest. Don't ask the question though if you do not want the answer. Personally, I ask loads of people for feedback as great stuff comes back and it's much cheaper than hiring a consultant.

COME ON!

- Here it is, your final cardio day of the course but not the final one of all time by any means.
- This should be just the start of a new lifestyle. You have been given an excellent grounding and this course should be a "stepping stone" to a full and healthy life.
- Change the time on your training program to 40 minutes for the run/jog. 20 minutes out and 20 minutes in. You should be looking to improve on your times consistently as you carry on with your program. Adjust the timings of your cardio session to fit in with your lifestyle. An hour is sufficient for a good level of health and fitness. Whichever cardio session you choose to do today, make it a brilliant one.

See you tomorrow for your final resistance session of this book.

#89. THE WAY AHEAD

Well, this book is rapidly coming to an end, but that doesn't mean that the healthy lifestyle finishes. You now have the grounding to carry this forward for the rest of your life.

Today we are looking at setting up your training plan for the immediate future. We will be devising a timetable that you will be in control of. We will be using the theories learnt on day #80 to move into a strength and power phase. Then we will put in an endurance phase, which the rep range is anything over 15 reps per set.

First you must decide on how many training sessions you are going to do in a normal week. This can be any number to suit your work and lifestyle. I have clients who train only on weekdays before they go to work using the weekends as rest days. 5 sessions a week is a great commitment but may not be possible or desirable for you. Split the sessions up if you can so that you alternate between a cardio-vascular session and a resistance session. My example is of a 4 day based training program. Remember, you decide on yours.

Week	Sun	Mon	Tue	Wed	Thu	Fri	Sat
1-6	Rest	Cardio	Strength 1	Rest	Cardio	Strength 2	Rest
7-12	Rest	Cardio	Power 1	Rest	Cardio	Power 2	Rest
13-18	Rest	Cardio	Endurance 1	Rest	Cardio	Endurance 2	Rest
19-24	Rest	Cardio	Build 1	Rest	Cardio	Build 2	Rest
25-30	Rest	Cardio	Strength 1	Rest	Cardio	Strength 2	Rest
31-36	Rest	Cardio	Power 1	Rest	Cardio	Power 2	Rest
37-42	Rest	Cardio	Endurance 1	Rest	Cardio	Endurance 2	Rest
43-48	Rest	Cardio	Build 1	Rest	Cardio	Build 2	Rest

A simple but effective yearly cycle, using the exercises in the sessions that you have already mastered.

As you get more experienced and learn new exercises, you can incorporate them into your program. Your body will become accustomed to the exercises that you are performing, which is why it is imperative that you change things from time to time. It is worth remembering that if you do what you always do, you will get what you've always got. If you want a change in body then you must change some of your training or eating plan.

The beauty of what we've done over the past 3 months is that our eating plan is varied and your allowance is constantly changing with your body weight and exercise output. The intensity of exercise is always changing, as you get stronger and fitter.

COME ON!

Big day today, there's plenty to do.

- Resistance Session 1.
- Devise your training plan for the next 6 months at least.
- Call yourself to action. Make that commitment to yourself because you truly deserve a fit and healthy body.

Before your graduation day tomorrow, just reflect (look back on the course if necessary) on just how much you've learnt and how far you've come in the last 12 weeks. You must be flexible enough by now to give yourself a big pat on the back. If not re-read #82 and #83.

See you tomorrow, sleep well you've deserved it.

#90. GRADUATION DAY

Congratulations, you've come a long way. 90 days of information, tips and a call to action that has changed the way you approach health and fitness. You are now armed with tons of valuable information that can be carried forward and used for the rest of your life.

Let's look back very quickly at some of the things you've now got up and running.

- Food diary so you know exactly how much you are taking on board.
- Method of calculating how much you are entitled to.
- Training program and plan that you are in control of.
- Vital nutritional information to help you to make the right food choices.

So what are your results of all this hard work? What we need to do is repeat the tests that you did at the beginning of the course and make comparisons. This is where we will see just how much you have changed in the 3 months together.

Evaluating the results.

The moment of truth has arrived and you have your results and comparisons. You will generally fall into one of these categories:

- **Chuffed to bits** - everything has worked better than you ever imagined. You're fitter, stronger and you're well on the way or have even reached your health and fitness goal. Very well done, you're amazing. But keep it up for life.

  Not many people reach this special place, so don't worry if you're not here yet. 3 months is a relatively short time to have got everything right.

- **Very pleased** - things are definitely happening. You feel better, fitter than before and are optimistic about the future. You know there's more to come and you have the drive to carry on. Very well done for making all the improvements. Stick with it you will soon be amazing.

This is where the majority of people find themselves after the first 3 months of a major lifestyle change. If you feel good now, just think how good you will feel after another 3 months. I told you at the start there are no quick fixes when it comes to health and fitness. Good luck with your progress.

- **Disappointed with the results** - all that hard work and nothing really happened. I'm still much the same as when I started.

  Unfortunately a few of you will be in this category. It's hand on heart time now. Did you really give it your best? Did you really push yourself on those cardio days (every time)? Did you eat sensibly and cruise with the booze etc? If the answer is not quite, or no then there's your explanation staring you straight between the eyes. But to be fair you would have known the results before you re-tested. If the answer was yes, you did give 100% then let's look at the options.

    - You might have an underlying medical condition that you are unaware of. A visit to your GP (Doctor) might be in order here.
    - You might have just over set your sights thinking that things happened at a quicker pace. The more you do, the easier it gets. - Stick with it and give it longer. Measure again after another 3 months but look at the positives you've got from the course.

COME ON! For the last time.

- Take the measurements and compare with day 1.
- Evaluate fairly your results (don't be too harsh with yourself).
- Email me with the results (through my website - www.stevehalls.co.uk)
- Finally think of 5 special people you know who would benefit from such a life-changing course. Show them how much you care about them (that you wish to see them around for much longer) and give them the perfect gift of life - The FBI, Come On!

Congratulations!

ABOUT STEVE HALLS

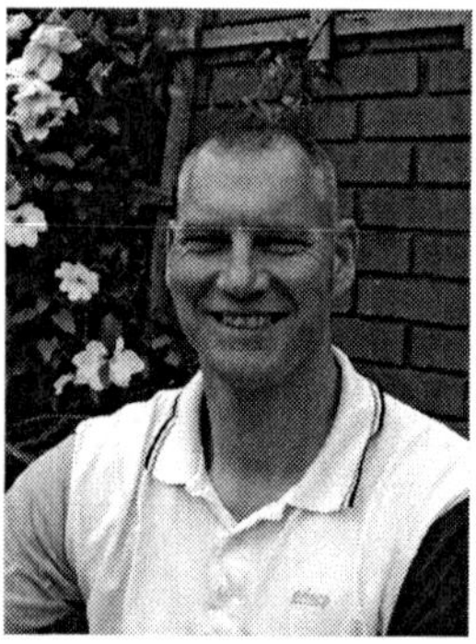

Born in Stoke-on-Trent England I attended schools in Caverswall and Cheadle in Staffordshire. I joined the British Army straight from school at a tender age of 16 where I served for more than 23 years. I attained the rank of Warrant Officer Class 1 before I left in 2000.

On leaving the Army, I took the Premier Diploma Course in Fitness Training and Sports Therapy. I gained experience working with such diverse groups as "British Military Fitness" and the ageing populations of which some had special medical issues such as Altzheimer's, Parkinson's and Dementia.

I Pride myself on making my training available for everyone, which has seen me work with many clients with MS, ME, Asthma and High Blood Pressure to name a few, along with active youngsters wishing to make the Forces their chosen career.

In 2004 I became the Fitness Director to the Academy of High Achievers. It was the meeting of such inspirational people in the Academy that inspired me to write my "Fit Body Initiative" eCourse. This is the Internet version of the book that is delivered to your inbox daily.

I am also an experienced keynote speaker delivering unique presentations on Health and Fitness throughout the country to corporate and private conferences.

My hobbies include folk singing and playing the guitar to any misguided person mad enough to want to listen. Also, for my positive stress input, I am a season ticket holder at Stoke City Football Club. For more information visit my website on www.stevehalls.co.uk

Printed in the United Kingdom
by Lightning Source UK Ltd.
121491UK00002B/247-327/P

9 781905 430086